Arthroscopic Surgery - New Perspectives
http://dx.doi.org/10.5772/intechopen.106447
Edited by William B. Stetson

Contributors
Adrian Todor, Alex Martusiewicz, Brett P. Wiater, Girinivasan Chellamuthu, Iffath Misbah, James Young Jin Lee, Jerome Michael Wiater, Joseph Choi, Margaret Jonas, Maxwell Li, Mazen Zamzam, Mihail-Lazar Mioc, Munis Ashraf, Petru Razvan Melinte, Radu Prejbeanu, William Wardell

First published in London, United Kingdom, 2024 by IntechOpen
IntechOpen is the global imprint of INTECHOPEN LIMITED, registered in England and Wales, registration number: 11086078, 5 Princes Gate Court, London, SW7 2QJ, United Kingdom

British Library Cataloguing-in-Publication Data
A catalogue record for this book is available from the British Library

Additional hard and PDF copies can be obtained from orders@intechopen.com

Arthroscopic Surgery - New Perspectives
Edited by William B. Stetson
p. cm.
Print ISBN 978-1-83768-882-1
Online ISBN 978-1-83768-883-8
eBook (PDF) ISBN 978-1-83768-884-5

For EU product safety concerns:
IN TECH d.o.o., Prolaz Marije Krucifikse Kozulić 3, 51000 Rijeka, Croatia,
info@intechopen.com or visit our website at intechopen.com.

Meet the editor

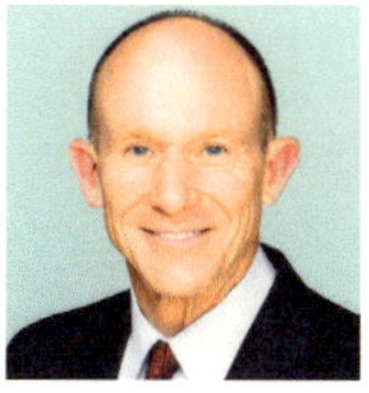

Dr. William B. Stetson is an award-winning orthopedic surgeon who is double board certified in orthopedic surgery and sports medicine. He is the Olympic team doctor for the USA men's and women's indoor volleyball teams. He is also a sports medicine, arthroscopy, and trauma specialist with expertise in the arthroscopic surgical reconstruction of complex shoulder, knee, elbow, and ankle injuries. Dr. Stetson has more than 25 years of teaching experience as a volunteer clinical professor of orthopedic surgery at Los Angeles County + USC Medical Center where he teaches the residents orthopedic surgery and arthroscopy. He is the author of more than 45 peer-reviewed publications and has more than 100 national and international presentations to his credit. He is the founder of Stetson Lee Orthopaedics and Sports Medicine, CA, USA, as well as the founder of Operation Arthroscopy (operationarthroscopy.org) and SurgTime (www.surgtime), a telesurgery platform.

Contents

Preface

Arthroscopic Surgery – New Perspectives provides current information on the cutting edge of arthroscopic surgical techniques for the shoulder and knee. The book addresses controversial topics in arthroscopy, presents the latest perspectives, and discusses how to deal with challenges. For the shoulder, chapters discuss the controversial topic of superior labrum anterior to posterior (SLAP) lesions and the latest arthroscopic techniques to address them. For rotator cuff tears, chapters examine the use of new biologics, augmentation with patches, tendon transfers, and balloon spacers.

I would like to thank all my co-authors who so generously donated their time and energy to this project and our editors and publishers at IntechOpen who kept us all on task and who were instrumental throughout the publication process.

William B. Stetson, M.D.
Associate Clinical Professor of Orthopaedic Surgery,
University of Southern California Keck School of Medicine,
Los Angeles, California, USA

Stetson Lee Orthopaedics and Sports Medicine,
CA, USA

Section 1

Shoulder

Chapter 1

Failure of SLAP Tear Repair and the Management of Long Head of Biceps Pathology

William Wardell, Margaret Jonas and Joesph Choi

Abstract

SLAP (superior labrum anterior-posterior) tears are a source of shoulder pain encountered by the orthopedic surgeon. These injuries are most frequently seen in young patients, notably overhead throwing athletes, in addition to older patients, commonly degenerative tears. Treatment of SLAP lesions initially consists of conservative measures including throwing rest, and physical therapy, especially in younger overhead throwing athletes. Operative treatment interventions include arthroscopic labral debridement alone, arthroscopic debridement with bicep anchor/labral repair, or arthroscopic debridement with biceps tenotomy or tenodesis. Patients over 40 years old are often treated with biceps tenotomy compared to tenodesis alone. Younger patients, especially overhead athletes less than 40 are typically treated with SLAP repair. Debate remains between the use of long head of biceps tenotomy compared to biceps tenodesis, either mini open (subpectoral) or arthroscopic (suprapectoral) tenodesis. This chapter will focus on the failure of SLAP repair and subsequent management, in addition to the role of biceps tenotomy versus tenodesis in the role of management of this pathology, either as the primary procedure or as an adjunct to repair.

Keywords: SLAP tear, biceps tenotomy, biceps tenodesis, SLAP repair, SLAP failure, superior labrum anterior posterior

1. Introduction

SLAP (superior labrum anterior-posterior) tears are a source of shoulder pain most frequently seen in young, overhead throwing athletes, as well as older patients, often seen as degenerative tears. These injuries are initially managed conservatively with rest, symptomatic treatment, and physical therapy. However, when conservative measures fail, operative treatment may be indicated. This chapter will focus on the failure of SLAP repairs as well as discuss the role of biceps tenotomy and tenodesis in the management of SLAP tears and long head of the biceps tendon pathology. Biceps tenotomy or tenodesis can be utilized either as the primary procedure or as an adjunct to SLAP repair.

2. SLAP (superior labrum anterior-posterior) tears

SLAP tears of the glenohumeral labrum are uncommon injuries most often seen in overhead throwing athletes. In the initial description by Andrews, it was found that most tears occur at the anterior-superior portion of the labrum in close proximity to the biceps insertion, and the long head of the biceps tendon is under increased stress in the throwing motion [1]. SLAP pathology is also associated with glenohumeral internal rotation deficit (GIRD), internal impingement, scapular dyskinesis and articular sided rotator cuff tears. Patient presentation is often delayed, with complaints of vague, nonspecific, deep shoulder pain. Throwing athletes will complain of decreased effectiveness and early fatigue [2, 3]. SLAP tears were initially classified by Snyder, which is the most commonly used classification system. The most common tear type, as defined by Snyder, was Type II, defined as fraying of the labrum with associated detachment of the biceps anchor [3]. The superior glenoid serves as the attachment point for the long head of the biceps, with insertion commonly occurring on the glenoid labrum. The biceps tendon anchor is the weakest point, leading to SLAP pathology [1]. The anatomy of this attachment is important in consideration of both the surgical treatment of SLAP lesions, and the post operative complications, including SLAP repair failure.

The diagnosis of a SLAP tear can be made with a combination of provocative physical examination maneuvers and imaging modalities. One option for advanced imaging is the magnetic resonance imaging (MRI) or magnetic resonance arthrogram (MRA). Studies have shown that MRA is better utilized for diagnosis of SLAP tear, as it can also be diagnostic for associated injuries including rotator cuff tear [4]. However, it is important to correlate imaging findings with patient history and clinical examination, as not all SLAP tears are symptomatic, or even require operative treatment. There are multiple studies that have evaluated the correlation of SLAP tear on MRI and impact on athletes, when they were asymptomatic. One such study found that there was no relationship between findings on imaging and likelihood of future symptoms in Major League Baseball players. However, this study did demonstrate that MRI findings were more common in players who pitched more innings, suggesting that these injuries are attributable to overuse and overhead throwing motion [5]. Additional studies suggest that there is a significant number of overhead athletes who have SLAP tears found on MRI but remain asymptomatic. For example, Stetson et al. published their MRI review of U.S. Olympic volleyball athletes, 46% of asymptomatic elite volleyball players had MRI evidence of SLAP tears or fraying but no history or complaints of shoulder problems. This suggests that non operative management can be a successful mainstay in these patients [6, 7]. This is extremely important to note due to the significantly poor outcomes with competitive overhead throwers who undergo surgical fixation of SLAP tears. Return to play in baseball players ranges from 7 to 62% [8–12].

Treatment of SLAP lesions initially consists of conservative measures including throwing rest and physical therapy. However increased level of overhead throwing may predispose athletes to failure of conservative treatment and physical therapy [13, 14]. A physical therapy regimen focuses to address underlying associated pathology including glenohumeral internal rotation deficit (GIRD) and internal impingement by addressing rotator cuff strengthening, posterior capsular stretching, and scapular stability. Operative treatment interventions include arthroscopic debridement alone, arthroscopic debridement with bicep anchor/labral repair, or arthroscopic debridement with biceps tenotomy or tenodesis.

The treatment algorithm for operative management of SLAP tears involves the patient's age, activity level, body habitus, and cosmetic expectations. Patients over age 40 are best treated with tenotomy of the long head of the biceps versus biceps tenodesis alone [6]. Younger patients, especially overhead-throwing athletes, are typically treated with SLAP repair and do not tolerate non operative treatment well [13, 15]. Surgical technique involves the use of suture anchors placed in the glenoid rim and configured optimally based on arthroscopic observation of labral tear [11, 16]. The most common adverse outcomes associated with SLAP repair are decreased rate of return to competitive sport and shoulder stiffness [2–4, 11, 13–16]. Shoulder stiffness is the most common complication following SLAP repair. Therefore, differentiating a type II SLAP tear from a meniscoid type of labrum, a normal sublabral foramen or variant is also critical to the success of the operation. Gobezie et al. showed that even among expert shoulder surgeons, interobserver and intraobserver reliability is poor (48%) in differentiating type II SLAP tears from normal variants or degenerative type I SLAP lesions. Arthroscopic repair of a normal variant can lead to loss of external rotation and alter normal throwing mechanics [17, 18]. SLAP repair failure is an additional complication seen.

3. SLAP tears repair failure

SLAP repair failure is defined as persistent shoulder pain with or without mechanical symptoms requiring additional treatment. SLAP repair failure is seen following arthroscopic repair with multiple potential etiologies. Common etiologies for SLAP repair failure include failure of the repair (which can be secondary to hardware failure of the suture anchors) or articular cartilage damage. SLAP repair is more often utilized and has shown to have greater effectiveness in patients who are younger than thirty-six years old [19]. Research shows that there are less complications and reported failures in patients who undergo tenodesis of the long head of the biceps and arthroscopic debridement, instead of repair [20–22]. Patients undergoing primary tenotomy or tenodesis of the long head of the biceps are typically older patients, however more recent studies suggest this as a viable treatment method in younger patients [15].

Complications and failure of SLAP repair are not infrequent and can cause significant exacerbation of symptoms in patients. SLAP repair failure is managed with either nonoperative management, revision SLAP repair, or repair revision to long head of the biceps tenodesis. Literature suggests that revision repair is well tolerated, however biceps tenodesis is better tolerated. Biceps tenodesis also demonstrates higher return to functional activity level [22]. The most prevalent complication following SLAP repair is post operative stiffness. In review of cases from the American Board of Orthopedic Surgery (ABOS) part II cases, it was noted that only 26.3% of patients reported absence of pain and only 13.1% of patients reported function as normal [23]. These findings help illustrate the impact of SLAP repair failure and the importance of preventing this complication. Numerous biomechanical studies have been performed with the goal of evaluating methods of SLAP repair. These studies address topics such as the number and location of suture anchors on the glenoid. A cadaveric study by Lehtinen found the optimal anchor position was found to be approximately a thirty-degree angle in relation to the articular surface, the anchor in this position provides the greatest glenoid bone stock to complete the repair [24]. In another cadaveric study focused on the configuration of suture anchors, they found that there is no biomechanical advantage to the placement of suture anchor anterior to the biceps anchor [25]. Prior studies have suggested that suture anchor placement anterior to the biceps anchor can lead to increased stiffness post operatively in SLAP repair [26].

The reason for SLAP repair failure is poorly understood, however there are multiple reasons hypothesized in the literature. One theory is that concomitant injuries lead to poor outcomes and the inability to return to sport, including rotator cuff tears. Ability to return to sport is also dependent upon position played, as there is significant evidence suggesting worse outcomes in baseball pitchers [9, 27, 28]. Additionally, SLAP repair has been shown to change pitching mechanics and yield diminished throwing performance highlighted by decreased velocity and inability to maintain command of their pitches. These altered mechanics were highlighted in a study by McLaughlin who found that pitchers who had undergone SLAP repair had decreased abduction, decreased external rotation, and forward trunk tilt [29]. In addition to patient factors, technical factors from surgery may also play a role in SLAP repair failure and poor patient outcomes. Review of the literature suggests that use of the trans-rotator cuff portal may lead to damage of the musculotendinous portion of the supraspinatus, which predisposes patients to decreased return to play and poor outcomes [17]. Using the trans rotator cuff portal, O'Brien et al. [30] reported a 44% return-to-sport rate and Cohen et al. [12] reported a 38% rate whereas Neri et al. [9] reported a 13% rate. Therefore, using a single anchor placed via a cannula through the rotator interval is recommended.

Studies also indicate that anchor location in SLAP repair can impact patient outcomes and may explain some of the biomechanical alterations seen including decreased external rotation. If the SLAP repair anchor is placed anteriorly, this can lead to loss of external rotation [27, 31] due to entrapment of the superior glenohumeral ligament and middle glenohumeral ligament causing an inadvertent small but statistically significant loss of external rotation [11, 32]. Furthermore, a biomechanical study of the peel-back mechanism of failure has shown no advantage to the placement of an anterior anchor [25].

Associated shoulder pathology may be another reason SLAP repairs fare so poorly. For example, baseball pitchers with partial rotator cuff tears at the time of SLAP repair have shown a lower rate of return to baseball. Neri et al. [9] reported that only 13% were able to return to base- ball, whereas Brockmeier et al. reported that 64% were able to return [11]. Partial articular-sided rotator cuff tears present a challenge to the surgeon. These need to be addressed with either debridement (<50% of the tendon involved) or repair (>50% of the tendon involved) either using a PASTA (partial articular supraspinatus tendon avulsion) repair technique, which is preferred in younger overhead athletes, or completing the tear and repairing it in older athletes [17].

The final technical point that may impact patient outcomes is the type of suture used to repair. Studies have demonstrated that mattress suture is able to better recreate the native labrum/glenoid interface, as well as provide a more robust fixation method when compared to a simple suture [33, 34]. Because of the prevalence of SLAP repair failure, additional research has been performed to evaluate the use of biceps tenodesis or tenotomy as primary treatment of SLAP repair.

4. Biceps tenodesis vs. biceps tenotomy

In addition to SLAP repair, SLAP pathology can be managed with long head of the biceps tenotomy or tenodesis. The clinical indications of long head of biceps tenotomy compared to biceps tenodesis are not universally agreed upon. Multiple techniques have been described for biceps tenodesis, and multiple studies have been performed to determine the clinical indications and utilization of tenodesis or tenotomy. Biceps tenodesis can be performed through an open or an arthroscopic approach, and the tendon may be anchored in a proximal suprapectoral (above the groove), suprapectoral (below the groove), or distal subpectoral position [1, 23, 24].

One popular method of all arthroscopic tenodesis is the "loop 'N' tack biceps tenodesis". This technique is a knotless, intra-articular, arthroscopy only technique [35]. The loop and tack technique involves standard arthroscopy positioning in either the lateral decubitus or beach chair position. A diagnostic arthroscopy is performed utilizing a standard posterior viewing portal and a standard anterior working portal is then made under direct visualization. Then, the surgeon passes a looped suture around the proximal portion of the long head of the biceps tendon and retrieves the loop through the anterior canula. The free end of the suture is placed through the loop to complete a luggage tag stitch (**Figure 1**). Utilizing a sharp arthroscopic tool, like the Bird Beak (Arthrex), the surgeon passes the free end of the suture through the biceps tendon to anchor to the humeral head. Then the proximal portion of the long head of the biceps is cut using either arthroscopic scissors, shaver, or radiofrequency device near the attachment point of the superior labrum. The free end of the suture is then anchored to the humerus at the superior border of the subscapularis and the most distal portion of the bicipital groove visualized (**Figure 2**). This can be done with the surgical anchor of the surgeon's preference [35].

Another option for repair is a mini-open subpectoral technique for biceps tenodesis utilizing all suture technique [36]. This subpectoral technique can utilize different fixation methods including a tenodesis screw, an all-suture anchor, or a cortical button for fixation of the biceps. The surgeon begins this technique by starting the patient in the beach chair position, utilizing a mechanical arm holder of the surgeon's choice for positioning of the operative extremity. Standard diagnostic arthroscopy is

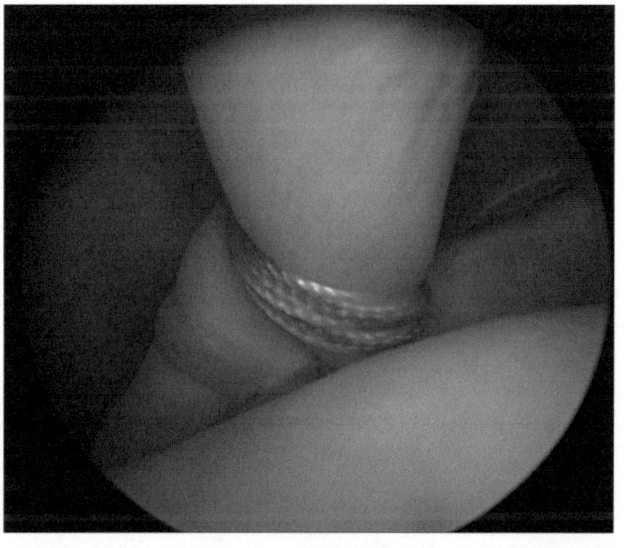

Figure 1.
Arthroscopic image of long head of the biceps tendon. Patient positioned in beach chair position, viewing from standard posterior shoulder portal. Loop suture has been secured around the biceps tendon. Suture is anchored to the humerus at the superior border of the subscapularis and the most distal portion of the bicipital groove.

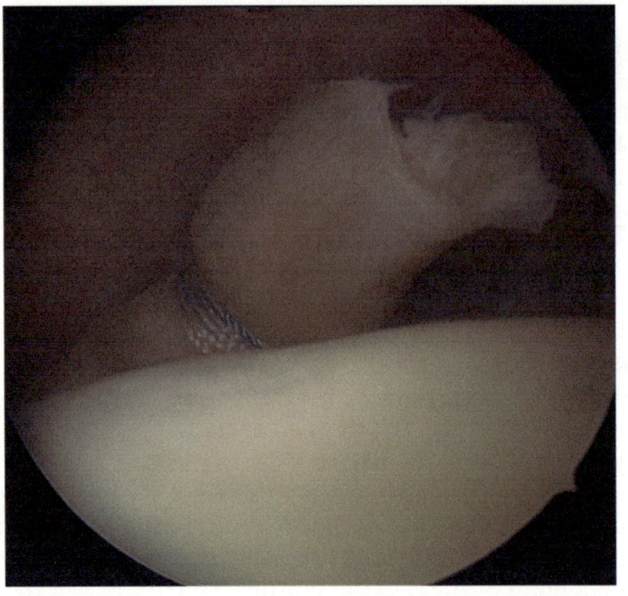

Figure 2.
Arthroscopic image of long head of the biceps tendon after completion of biceps tenodesis with tenotomy utilizing arthroscopic scissor. Patient positioned in beach chair position, viewing from standard posterior shoulder portal.

performed with a standard posterior viewing portal and a standard anterior working portal, made under direct visualization. Tenotomy of the pathologic long head of the biceps is performed using either arthroscopic scissors, radiofrequency device, or shaver. Attention is then turned distally to the subpectoral bicipital groove. The arm is abducted and externally rotated to expose the pectoralis major tendon; a longitudinal skin incision is made distal to this. The coracobrachialis, biceps and pectoralis are identified. The long head of the biceps is palpated after retraction of the pectoralis major tendon. A clamp is then placed around the long head of the biceps tendon and the free end of the tendon is then delivered through the skin incision [36]. At this point multiple different fixation devices have been described including the all-suture anchor technique, tenodesis interference screw, and cortical button [36, 37]. There is no generalized consensus as to which of these techniques yields the best results.

Research on this topic comparing the use of the interference screw versus all suture anchor showed that the two options were equivalent in both ultimate failure load and stiffness [38]. There is no general consensus regarding which tenodesis technique leads to the best outcomes; both all-arthroscopic biceps tenodesis and open subpectoral biceps tenodesis are viable treatment methods for management of pathology of the long head of the biceps [9].

Conversely, biceps tenotomy is also an option in management of long head of the biceps pathology. The patient is positioned in either the beach chair or lateral decubitus position, based on surgeon comfort and preference. Pathologic long head of the biceps tendon is visualized through the standard posterior portal (**Figure 3**). Tenotomy is best achieved using arthroscopic scissors, shaver, or radiofrequency device near the attachment point of the superior labrum, depending on surgeon preference (**Figure 4**). Meeks reported high patient satisfaction with reported 13% rate of cosmetic deformity in patients who underwent biceps tenotomy. These results suggest that tenotomy alone is a viable alternative surgical management [39]. Other concerns with biceps tenotomy include decreased supination function and muscle cramping. This study demonstrates similar results regarding biceps cramping, 20%, when compared to other tenotomy evaluations [39]. With this alternative in treatment, multiple studies exist comparing biceps tenotomy and tenodesis.

Biceps tenotomy compared to tenodesis has been a frequently studied topic. According to multiple review articles and meta-analysis, tenotomy is more likely to result in cosmetic deformity, Popeye deformity, and muscle cramping (although cramping is not obviated by performing tenodesis). Additionally, tenotomy has also shown decreased functional scores and diminished supination strength [40, 41]. Additional meta-analysis demonstrates there is increased incidence of cosmetic deformity and post operative cramping with tenotomy, however there are no functional differences noted between tenotomy and tenodesis of the long head of the biceps [42]. Tenotomy is best utilized in older, overweight patients, with less functional demand, and less concern for cosmesis [41]. Tenodesis is often reserved for younger, higher functional demand, and less likely to tolerate Popeye deformity [41]. Tenodesis can be performed in patients best suited for tenotomy, however there may be no clinical benefit in this patient population.

As discussed above, tenodesis can be performed all arthroscopically, using the loop and tack technique, or using a mini open technique using a tenodesis interference screw, tightrope with cortical button, or suture/suture anchor utilizing an onlay technique. These techniques have been studied, with no general consensus. Studies demonstrate favorable results with use of these tenodesis techniques, especially in management of SLAP repairs, however there is no general consensus.

Newer research advocates for the use of tenodesis in the treatment of SLAP repairs in younger patients, especially those who participate in overhead throwing activities. The study by Pogorzelski evaluated the use of biceps tenodesis utilizing biceps

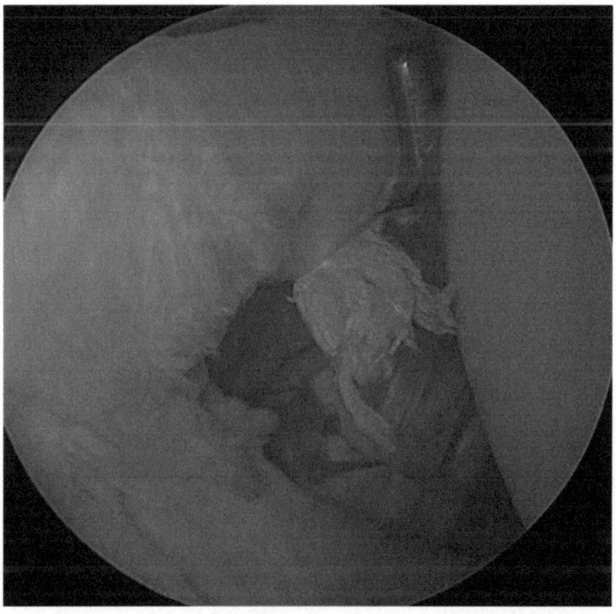

Figure 3.
Arthroscopic image of diseased long head of the biceps tendon with probe placed around tendon. Patient positioned in lateral decubitus position, viewing from standard posterior shoulder portal.

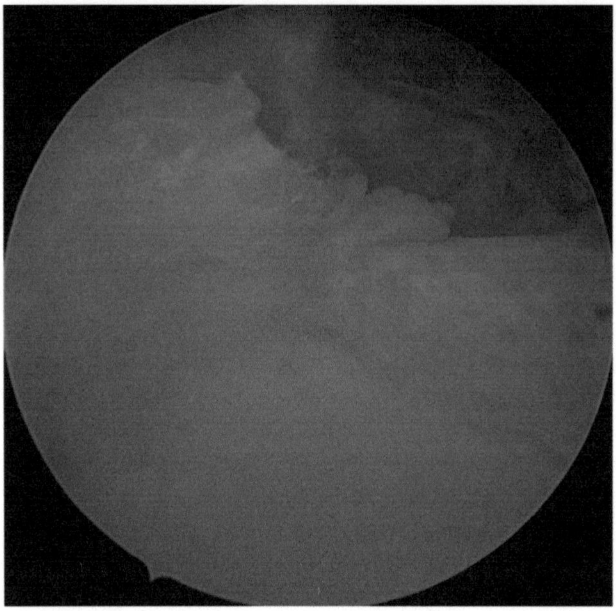

Figure 4.
Arthroscopic image of long head of the superior glenoid labrum and biceps anchor after completion of biceps tenotomy with arthroscopic shave. Patient positioned in lateral decubitus position, viewing from standard posterior shoulder portal.

tenotomy with radiofrequency device followed by mini open subpectoral biceps tenodesis with utilization of tenodesis screw. Results demonstrated patients had significant improvement in American Shoulder Elbow Society Scores (ASES) and a 90% rate of return to preoperative level of function, including return to sports and overhead activities [15]. Additional review demonstrates comparable return to sport in patients undergoing SLAP repair compared to biceps tenodesis, although these results do not account for activity, including overhead throwing versus non overhead throwing athletes [43]. Other attempted treatment modalities in this population includes repair of the SLAP tear with concomitant biceps tenodesis, however these results show that these patients experience worse outcomes in comparison to patients undergoing primary repair or biceps tenodesis in isolation [44]. This may demonstrate the role of biceps tenodesis in younger, overhead throwing athletes. Given the complication rates and failures noted in SLAP repair, more studies are necessary to evaluate the role of biceps tenodesis compared to SLAP repair.

5. Conclusions

SLAP (superior labrum anterior-posterior) tears are a source of shoulder pain most frequently seen in young, overhead throwing, patients, as well as older patients, degenerative tears. SLAP lesions and concomitant shoulder pathology is best diagnosed using advanced imaging including magnetic resonance imaging (MRI) and magnetic resonance arthrogram (MRA). Treatment of SLAP lesions initially consists of conservative measures including throwing rest, in younger, overhead throwing athletes and physical therapy. Operative treatment interventions include arthroscopic debridement alone, arthroscopic debridement with bicep anchor/labral repair, or arthroscopic debridement with biceps tenotomy or tenodesis. Patients over 40 are best treated with biceps tenotomy vs. tenodesis alone. Younger patients, especially overhead athletes less than 40 are typically treated with SLAP repair. There is a high incidence of SLAP repair failure in competitive overhead athletes that is multifactorial in nature, secondary to patient characteristics and surgical technique. There remains debate between the use of long head of biceps tenotomy compared to biceps tenodesis, either mini open (subpectoral) or arthroscopic tenodesis. Tenotomy is best utilized in older, overweight patients, with less functional demand, and less concern for cosmesis. Tenodesis is often reserved for younger, higher functional demand, and less likely to tolerate Popeye deformity.

Conflict of interest

The authors declare no conflict of interest.

Author details

William Wardell[1], Margaret Jonas[2]* and Joesph Choi[1]

1 Guthrie/Robert Packer Hospital, Sayre, PA, United States of America

2 Christus Health, Corpus Christi, TX, United States of America

*Address all correspondence to: margaret.jonas@guthrie.org

References

[1] Andrews JR, Carson WG Jr, McLeod WD. Glenoid labrum tears related to the long head of the biceps. The American Journal of Sports Medicine. 1985;**13**(5):337-341. DOI: 10.1177/036354658501300508

[2] Kim TK, Queale WS, Cosgarea AJ, McFarland EG. Clinical features of the different types of SLAP lesions: An analysis of one hundred and thirty-nine cases. The Journal of Bone and Joint Surgery. American Volume. 2003;**85**(1):66-71

[3] Snyder SJ, Banas MP, Karzel RP. An analysis of 140 injuries to the superior glenoid labrum. Journal of Shoulder and Elbow Surgery. 1995;**4**(4):243-248. DOI: 10.1016/s1058-2746(05)80015-1

[4] Stetson WB, Templin K. The crank test, the O'Brien test, and routine magnetic resonance imaging scans in the diagnosis of labral tears. The American Journal of Sports Medicine. 2002;**30**(6):806-809

[5] Lesniak BP, Baraga MG, Jose J, Smith MK, Cunningham S, Kaplan LD. Glenohumeral findings on magnetic resonance imaging correlate with innings pitched in asymptomatic pitchers. The American Journal of Sports Medicine. 2013;**41**(9):2022-2027

[6] Connor PM, Banks DM, Tyson AB, Coumas JS, D'Alessandro DF. Magnetic resonance imaging of the asymptomatic shoulder of overhead athletes: A 5-year follow-up study. The American Journal of Sports Medicine. 2003;**31**(5):724-727

[7] Stetson WB, Goldhaber NH, Powell SE, Lee CS. Magnetic resonance imaging findings in asymptomatic elite overhead athletes. Arthroscopy. 2017;**33**:58-59

[8] Fedoriw WW, Ramkumar P, McCulloch PC, Lintner DM. Return to play after treatment of superior labral tears in professional baseball players. The American Journal of Sports Medicine. 2014;**42**(5):1155-1160

[9] Neri BR, ElAttrache NS, Owsley KC, Mohr K, Yocum LA. Outcome of type II superior labral anterior posterior repairs in elite overhead athletes: Effect of concomitant partial-thickness rotator cuff tears. The American Journal of Sports Medicine. 2011;**39**(1):114-120

[10] Gilliam BD, Douglas L, Fleisig GS, Aune KT, Mason KA, Dugas JR, et al. Return to play and outcomes in baseball players after superior labral anterior-posterior repairs. The American Journal of Sports Medicine. 2018;**46**(1):109-115

[11] Brockmeier SF, Voos JE, Williams RJ 3rd, Altchek DW, Cordasco FA, Allen AA. Hospital for special surgery sports medicine and shoulder service. outcomes after arthroscopic repair of type-II SLAP lesions. The Journal of Bone and Joint Surgery. American Volume. 2009;**91**(7):1595-1603

[12] Cohen DB, Coleman S, Drakos MC, Allen AA, O'Brien SJ, Altchek DW, et al. Outcomes of isolated type II SLAP lesions treated with arthroscopic fixation using a bioabsorbable tack. Arthroscopy. 2006;**22**(2):136-142

[13] Jang SH, Seo JG, Jang HS, Jung JE, Kim JG. Predictive factors associated with failure of nonoperative treatment of superior labrum anterior-posterior tears. Journal of Shoulder and Elbow Surgery. 2016;**25**(3):428-434

[14] Knesek M, Skendzel JG, Dines JS, Altchek DW, Allen AA, Bedi A.

Diagnosis and management of superior labral anterior posterior tears in throwing athletes. The American Journal of Sports Medicine. 2013;**41**(2):444-460

[15] Pogorzelski J, Horan MP, Hussain ZB, Vap A, Fritz EM, Millett PJ. Subpectoral biceps tenodesis for treatment of isolated type II SLAP lesions in a young and active population. Arthroscopy. 2018;**34**(2):371-376

[16] Ek ET, Shi LL, Tompson JD, Freehill MT, Warner JJ. Surgical treatment of isolated type II superior labrum anterior-posterior (SLAP) lesions: Repair versus biceps tenodesis. Journal of Shoulder and Elbow Surgery. 2014;**23**(7):1059-1065

[17] Stetson WB, Polinsky S, Morgan SA, Strawbridge J, Carcione J. Arthroscopic repair of type II SLAP lesions in overhead athletes. Arthroscopy Techniques. 2019;**8**(7):e781-e792

[18] Gobezie R, Zurakowski D, Lavery K, Millett PJ, Cole BJ, Warner JJ. Analysis of interobserver and intraobserver variability in the diagnosis and treatment of SLAP tears using the Snyder classification. The American Journal of Sports Medicine. 2008;**36**:1373-1379

[19] Provencher MT, McCormick F, Dewing C, McIntire S, Solomon D. A prospective analysis of 179 type 2 superior labrum anterior and posterior repairs: Outcomes and factors associated with success and failure. The American Journal of Sports Medicine. 2013;**41**(4):880-886

[20] Werner BC, Evans CL, Holzgrefe RE, Tuman JM, Hart JM, Carson EW, et al. Arthroscopic suprapectoral and open subpectoral biceps tenodesis: A comparison of minimum 2-year clinical outcomes. The American Journal of Sports Medicine. 2014;**42**(11):2583-2590

[21] Denard PJ, Lädermann A, Parsley BK, Burkhart SS. Arthroscopic biceps tenodesis compared with repair of isolated type II SLAP lesions in patients older than 35 years. Orthopedics. 2014;**37**(3):e292-e297

[22] Nadeem IM, Vancolen S, Horner NS, Leroux T, Alolabi B, Khan M. Management of failed SLAP repair: A systematic review. HSS Journal. 2020;**16**(3):261-271

[23] Weber SC, Martin DF, Seiler JG 3rd, Harrast JJ. Superior labrum anterior and posterior lesions of the shoulder: Incidence rates, complications, and outcomes as reported by American Board of Orthopedic Surgery. Part II candidates. The American Journal of Sports Medicine. 2012;**40**(7):1538-1543

[24] Lehtinen JT, Tingart MJ, Apreleva M, Ticker JB, Warner JJ. Anatomy of the superior glenoid rim. Repair of superior labral anterior to posterior tears. The American Journal of Sports Medicine. 2003;**31**(2):257-260

[25] Morgan RJ, Kuremsky MA, Peindl RD, Fleischli JE. A biomechanical comparison of two suture anchor configurations for the repair of type II SLAP lesions subjected to a peel-back mechanism of failure. Arthroscopy. 2008;**24**(4):383-388

[26] Yoneda M, Hirooka A, Saito S, Yamamoto T, Ochi T, Shino K. Arthroscopic stapling for detached superior glenoid labrum. Journal of Bone and Joint Surgery. British Volume (London). 1991;**73**(5):746-750

[27] Chalmers PN, Erickson BJ, Verma NN, D'Angelo J, Romeo AA. Incidence and return to play after biceps tenodesis in professional baseball players. Arthroscopy. 2018;**34**(3):747-751

[28] Gorantla K, Gill C, Wright RW. The outcome of type II SLAP repair: A systematic review. Arthroscopy. 2010;**26**(4):537-545

[29] Laughlin WA, Fleisig GS, Scillia AJ, Aune KT, Cain EL Jr, Dugas JR. Deficiencies in pitching biomechanics in baseball players with a history of superior labrum anterior-posterior repair. The American Journal of Sports Medicine. 2014;**42**(12):2837-2841

[30] O'Brien SJ, Allen AA, Coleman SH, et al. The trans- rotator cuff approach to SLAP lesions: Technical aspects for repair and a clinical follow-up of 31 patients at a minimum of 2 years. Arthroscopy. 2002;**18**:372-377

[31] Kartus J, Ejerhed L, Funck E, Köhler K, Sernert N, Karlsson J. Arthroscopic and open shoulder stabilization using absorbable implants. A clinical and radiographic comparison of two methods. Knee Surgery, Sports Traumatology, Arthroscopy. 1998;**6**(3):181-188

[32] McCulloch PC, Andrews WJ, Alexander J, Brekke A, Duwani S, Noble P. The effect on external rotation of an anchor placed anterior to the biceps in type 2 SLAP repairsina cadaveric throwing model. Arthroscopy. 2013;**29**:18-24

[33] Domb BG, Ehteshami JR, Shindle MK, Gulotta L, Zoghi-Moghadam M, MacGillivray JD, et al. Biomechanical comparison of 3 suture anchor configurations for repair of type II SLAP lesions. Arthroscopy. 2007;**23**(2):135-140

[34] Dines JS, Elattrache NS. Horizontal mattress with a knotless anchor to better recreate the normal superior labrum anatomy. Arthroscopy. 2008;**24**(12):1422-1425

[35] Hammarstedt JE, Rinaldi J, Guth JJ, Akhavan S. The loop 'N' tack biceps Tenodesis: An all-arthroscopic, intra-articulartechnique.ArthroscopyTechniques. 2020;**9**(12):e1899-e1902

[36] Lacheta L, Imhoff AB, Siebenlist S, Scheiderer B. Subpectoral biceps tenodesis: All-suture anchor Onlay technique. Arthroscopy Techniques. 2020;**9**(5):e651-e655

[37] Kennedy NI, Godin JA, Ferrari MB, Sanchez G, Cinque ME, Hussain ZB, et al. Subpectoral biceps tenodesis: Interference screw and cortical button fixation. Arthroscopy Techniques. 2017;**6**(4):e1415-e1420

[38] Chiang FL, Hong CK, Chang CH, Lin CL, Jou IM, Su WR. Biomechanical comparison of all-suture anchor fixation and interference screw technique for subpectoral biceps tenodesis. Arthroscopy. 2016;**32**(7):1247-1252

[39] Meeks BD, Meeks NM, Froehle AW, Wareing E, Bonner KF. Patient satisfaction after biceps tenotomy. Orthopaedic Journal of Sports Medicine. 2017;**5**(5):2325967117707737

[40] Liu H, Song X, Liu P, Yu H, Zhang Q, Guo W. Clinical outcomes of arthroscopic tenodesis versus tenotomy for long head of the biceps tendon lesions: A systematic review and meta-analysis of randomized clinical trials and cohort studies. Orthopaedic Journal of Sports Medicine. 2021;**9**(4):2325967121993805

[41] Hsu AR, Ghodadra NS, Provencher MT, Lewis PB, Bach BR. Biceps tenotomy versus tenodesis: A review of clinical outcomes and biomechanical results. Journal of Shoulder and Elbow Surgery. 2011;**20**(2):326-332

[42] Gurnani N, van Deurzen DF, Janmaat VT, van den Bekerom MP. Tenotomy or tenodesis for pathology of the long head of the biceps brachii: A systematic review and meta-analysis. Knee Surgery, Sports Traumatology, Arthroscopy. 2016;**24**(12):3765-3771

[43] Abdul-Rassoul H, Defazio M, Curry EJ, Galvin JW, Li X. Return to sport after the surgical treatment of superior labrum anterior to posterior tears: A systematic review. Orthopaedic Journal of Sports Medicine. 2019;7(5):2325967119841892

[44] Chalmers PN, Monson B, Frank RM, Mascarenhas R, Nicholson GP, Bach BR Jr, et al. Combined SLAP repair and biceps tenodesis for superior labral anterior-posterior tears. Knee Surgery, Sports Traumatology, Arthroscopy. 2016;**24**(12):3870-3876

Chapter 2

Treatment of Rotator Cuff Tears: New Modalities and Innovations

James Young Jin Lee, Mazen Zamzam, Maxwell Li, Alex Martusiewicz, Brett P. Wiater and Jerome Michael Wiater

Abstract

Although frequently performed, rotator cuff repair carries a not insignificant failure rate. A number of studies including biomechanical and clinical studies have attempted to identify factors affecting rotator cuff repair and healing. Poor prognostic factors likely include age, fatty atrophy of rotator cuff muscles, large tear size, chronicity, and smoking. Recent rotator cuff tear research has been devoted to addressing both biologic and structural concerns of repair. Adjuvant repair techniques aimed at improving biology have emerged, and many are now clinically available and include biologic patch augmentation, bone marrow aspirate, platelet-rich plasma, and utilizing local bone marrow egress. Novel structural techniques have been developed to augment, alter, or replicate the structural properties of rotator cuff, particularly in the setting of irreparable rotator cuff tears. These include subacromial balloon spacers, tendon transfers, superior capsular reconstruction, anterior cable reconstruction, bursal acromial reconstruction, and biologic tuberoplasty. This chapter will examine these novel biological and structural techniques and review available clinical outcomes.

Keywords: rotator cuff repair, patch augmentation, biologics, novel rotator cuff reconstruction techniques, shoulder arthroscopy

1. Introduction

The prevalence of rotator cuff tears within the general population is estimated to be approximately 22.1% [1]. It is the most common source of shoulder pain and disability [2, 3]. As a result, arthroscopic rotator cuff repair is one of the most frequently performed orthopedic procedures [4, 5].

The most common complaint of a patient with a torn rotator cuff is pain [5]. In a study by Itoi et al. 87.9% of patients reported shoulder pain as the reason for the visit, and 10.8% reported pain and muscle weakness [6]. First-line treatments commonly include nonsteroidal anti-inflammatory (NSAIDs), corticosteroid injections, and physical therapy.

Although frequently performed, rotator cuff repair carries a not insignificant failure rate. Retear rates may range from 20% to 70% [7–11]. A number of studies including biomechanical and clinical studies have attempted to identify factors affecting rotator cuff repair and healing. Poor prognostic factors likely include age, fatty atrophy of rotator cuff muscles, large tear size, chronicity, and smoking.

Recent rotator cuff tear research has been devoted to addressing both biological and structural concerns of repair. Adjuvant repair techniques aimed at improving biology have emerged, and many are now clinically available and include biologic patch augmentation, bone marrow aspirate, platelet-rich plasma, and utilizing local bone marrow egress. Novel structural techniques have been developed to augment, alter, or replicate the structural properties of rotator cuff, particularly in the setting of irreparable rotator cuff tears. These include subacromial balloon spacers, tendon transfers, and superior capsular reconstruction (SCR), anterior cable reconstruction (ACR), bursal acromial reconstruction (BAR), and biologic tuberoplasty. This chapter will examine these novel biological and structural techniques and will review the available clinical outcomes.

2. Biologic augmentation of rotator cuff repair: An evolving field

Primary rotator cuff repair itself continues to evolve. Recent advancements in repair techniques and materials have allowed for continued improvement in time-zero fixation. These include various anchor types, suture materials, stitch configurations, and tissue penetrating devices [12]. However, retear rates after rotator cuff repair remain high, ranging from 20% to 40% at 2 years [11, 13–16]. As such, tendon repair augmentation methods have been proposed to provide a biological scaffold for mechanical stability and long-term incorporation by providing a porous structure onto which collagen can migrate. The utilization of a mechanical augmentation patch dates back to 1986. Ozaki et al. utilized Teflon felt to augment rotator cuff repair [17].

Cuff augmentation can be utilized in several different ways. It can be utilized as a mechanical interposition graft to bridge the gap between the tendon and bone when the tendon does not reach the footprint in the setting of a retracted, irreparable tear [9–11]. Second, an augmentation patch can be applied on the bursal side of the repair in an "on-lay" fashion [18]. Third, biologic grafts can be interposed between the tendon and the bone with the goal of promoting soft tissue integration and subsequent robust healing.

Many types of grafts are available for use in the market currently. These include synthetic, xenograft, allograft, or autograft patches. Several early studies utilized xenograft small intestine submucosal graft, which revealed high rates of repair failure as well as a profound inflammatory response and led to poor clinical outcomes [19, 20]. As such, utilization of small intestine submucosal graft has largely been abandoned. The simple on-lay of reconstituted bovine collagen implant (REGENETEN, Smith, and Nephews) impregnated with growth factors has been shown to significantly increase tendon thickness in the setting of partial thickness rotator cuff tears as seen on MRI at 2 years. These patients also reported improved clinical outcomes. Despite these promising early results on the REGENETEN patch, high-level comparative studies are needed to draw conclusions on its superiority over standard repair or other augmentation methods (**Figure 1**) [21].

A randomized controlled trial of 92 patients utilizing an acellular porcine dermal matrix scaffold in small to medium rotator cuff tears showed improved constant and strength scores compared to the nonbiologically augmented group. This evidence suggests an accelerated return to function without any graft-specific complications [22]. Similar results were seen in a randomized controlled trial of 112 patients with large

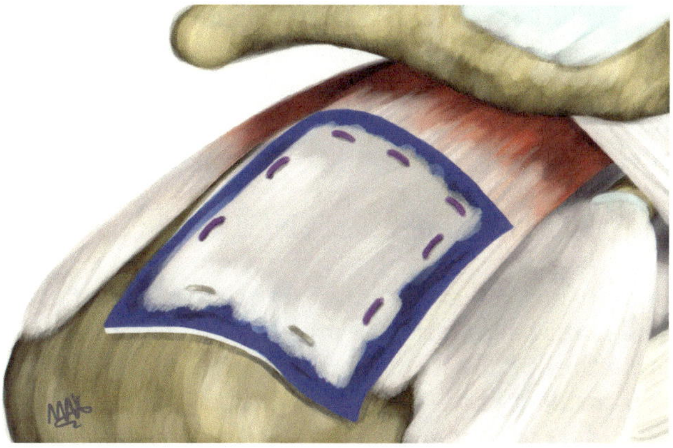

Figure 1.
Schematic of reconstituted bovine collagen implant (REGENETEN, Smith, and Nephews) used in an on-lay fashion to augment rotator cuff repair.

to massive rotator cuff using a synthetic 3D collagen scaffold augmentation. This study showed significantly higher 6-month UCLA and constant scores, suggesting an earlier return to function, although no difference was found at the final follow-up of 28 months [23].

The most utilized form of allograft rotator cuff augmentation is an acellular dermal allograft. This graft is composed of type I collagen processed to remove donor cells while preserving the extracellular matrix. Several acellular dermal allografts are available and have been utilized in orthopedic surgery and plastic surgery for decades. In biomechanical studies, allograft augmentation utilized in an on-lay fashion on top of a repair likely increases the load to failure in rotator cuff tendon repairs [24]. In vivo studies have demonstrated that the removal of cellular components allows infiltration of fibroblasts, tenocytes, and vascular tissues while causing minimal host inflammation [25, 26]. High porosity seen in new generations of "open matrix" dermal allografts may allow for deeper penetration of mesenchymal cells, leading to fibroplasia. Clinically, a prospective randomized study of 42 patients showed higher rates of the intact cuff in the on-lay acellular dermal patch augmentation group compared with the control group (85% vs. 40%) with higher American shoulder and elbow surgeons (ASES) and Constant scores at 2 years [27]. Autograft such as tensor fascia lata has also been utilized for rotator cuff augmentation with superior constant scores compared to partial repairs in a cohort study of 48 patients at minimum 7-year follow-up [28].

The use of biological and structural augmentation is an emerging solution to enhance healing in rotator cuff surgery. Various options are clinically available, and the popularity of these techniques continues to grow. Although promising data is emerging, further high-level comparative studies are necessary to define the indications, efficacy, and value.

3. Superior capsular reconstruction: Indications, techniques, and outcomes

SCR is a surgical procedure performed in the setting of irreparable cuff tears. The goal of SCR is to restore the stability of the shoulder joints, thereby re-establishing the mechanical fulcrum of the joint to the level of the glenohumeral articulation and potentially improving the force couple of the remaining rotator cuff tendons. Originally, SCR was described using a fascia lata autograft patch [29]. SCR is indicated for patients with a nonarthritic glenohumeral joint and a functional deltoid in the setting of an irreparable rotator cuff tendon (RCT) tear [29]. Patients with an intact subscapularis tendon also show improved outcomes compared to subscapularis deficient shoulders [30]. Ideally, patients should have a repairable or intact subscapularis when undergoing an SCR [30, 31].

The most commonly utilized and studied grafts are fascia lata autograft and extracellular dermal matrix allograft. The procedure can also be performed either arthroscopically or in the open, with sutures and anchors being placed either before or after the placement of the graft [32]. The original SCR technique involves an arthroscopic procedure to be done using a fascia lata autograft that is attached medially to the glenoid using two titanium suture anchors and laterally to the greater tuberosity using double-row techniques and suture bridge. The graft is stabilized with a side-to-side suture posteriorly to the residual infraspinatus and anteriorly to the subscapularis or residual anterior-superior tendon [29].

SCR outcomes are variable. The original authors of the technique involved 24 shoulders who underwent SCR with a fascia lata [29]. Thirty-four months after surgery, patients demonstrated improved active abduction and external rotation as well as improved ASES scores [29]. Denard et al. studied 59 patients who had an SCR and showed improvements in forward flexion, external rotation, VAS, and ASES scores [33]. Unfortunately, 11 (18.6%) of patients in the study underwent a revision procedure, including seven of them undergoing reverse shoulder arthroplasties [9]. More recently, Pennington published outcomes with 86 patients who underwent SCR with a dermal allograft and demonstrated significant improvements in ASES and VAS scores after 16–28 months [34].

The rehabilitation protocol for patients who undergo a SCR is similar to those who also undergo massive rotator cuff repairs. For the first 4 to 6 weeks, postoperatively, patients are placed in a sling with an abduction pillow. Generally, progressive range of motion (ROM) exercises when the wedge is removed at 4–6 weeks postoperatively. Most surgeons then have patients begin strengthening exercises at 12 weeks postoperatively, but a subset starts as early as the 8-week mark (**Figure 2**) [35].

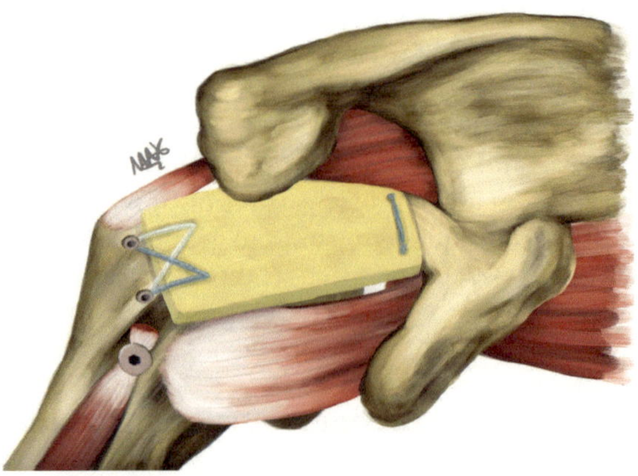

Figure 2.
Schematic of a SCR done using dermal cellular allograft fixed using suture anchors (note: long head of biceps tenodesed).

4. The subacromial balloon spacer for irreparable rotator cuff tears

Approximately half of all patients diagnosed with a torn rotator cuff undergo a surgical repair [36]. A subset of these patients are found either preoperatively or intraoperatively to have tears that are too large and retracted to perform a primary repair. As stated earlier, graft augmentation or SCR may be considered by both to be technically difficult to perform and may not be the ideal choice for lower-demand individuals. Also, there is some evidence that procedures that utilize grafts may negatively affect the outcomes of subsequent reverse shoulder arthroplasty (RSA) [37]. In lieu of this, the InSpace subacromial balloon (Stryker, USA) spacer was developed in 2010 [37] and was food and drug administration (FDA)-approved in 2021. The device consists of a saline-filled biodegradable balloon which is inserted between the humeral head and the acromion [38]. After arthroscopic insertion in the subacromial space, the InSpace balloon is insufflated with a recommended volume of saline proportional to the implant size selected. The outer material of the balloon is made of a copolymer designed to degrade in 12 months 7. It is theorized that a pseudocapsule remains after it degrades to help maintain the balloon effect. Currently, it is indicated in patients with massive (>5 cm) irreparable tears involving two or more tendons with a functional deltoid, little to no glenohumeral joint osteoarthritis, and preserved passive range of motion on examination. Similar SCR, the goal of the subacromial balloon is to restore the acromio-humeral interval and thereby re-establishing the normal mechanic of the shoulder during elevation. A theoretical advantage is that it may also reduce friction between tissue planes and potentially result in less early postoperative pain [38, 39].

While the InSpace subacromial balloon spacer is a novel device, it has already been implanted in approximately 29,000 patients internationally. However, current research is limited, and further studies are needed to evaluate its efficacy and safety. Nevertheless, the InSpace subacromial balloon spacer holds great promise in the management of irreparable rotator cuff tears, particularly in patients who are not suitable for more complex procedures (**Figure 3**).

Given earlier availability of the implant in Europe, international studies provide more data on postoperative outcomes of the surgical procedure. Gervasi et al. [40] showed that pain score improvement was found as early as 1 week postoperatively,

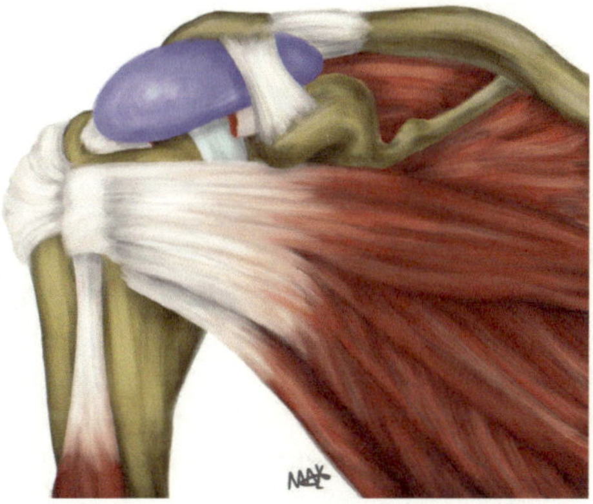

Figure 3.
Schematic diagram of InSPACE balloon inserted in the subacromial space.

and strength improvement 18 months postoperatively. Constant scores increased from 31.9 to 69.8 at 1 year follow-ups, demonstrating improvements in function, and mobility. More recently, a level 1 randomized controlled study emerged from the United States to evaluate the balloon over the course of 2 years. Participants underwent a partial tendon repair or an InSpace balloon insertion. ASES scores improved for both groups; however, a larger increase was noted for the InSpace group (46.22 vs. 42.53) [41]. InSpace implants also demonstrated functional and patient-reported outcomes comparable to partial repair of irreparable massive rotator cuff tears with intact subscapularis [41]. The InSpace device group demonstrated an earlier recovery based on improvements in ASES, WORC, and constant scores [41]. The range of motion measurements was also superior [41]. After the degradation of the implant, a 2-year follow-up demonstrated maintained clinical improvement.

Although the results of Hazra et al. are promising, other studies challenge this. A multicenter double-blinded randomized controlled trial (START:REACTS) in the United Kingdom showed less desirable outcomes [42]. This study randomized patients to debridement alone vs. debridement and subacromial balloon spacer insertion. This study was prematurely halted due to statistically greater improvement in the debridement alone group. While considered one of the emerging techniques for massive irreparable rotator cuff tears, the technique is considered controversial due to the conflicting data from the two high-level randomized controlled trials. Although approved for use by the FDA, further high-quality research is necessary to establish the role of the subacromial balloon spacer in treating irreparable rotator cuff tears.

Relative indications for use:

1. Irreparable symptomatic full-thickness massive rotator cuff tear:

    a. Measuring 5 cm or greater in diameter

    b. Involving two or more tendons

3. Functional deltoid muscle and preserved passive range of motion on physical examination

4. Absence of severe glenohumeral arthritis (Hamada grade 3 or greater)

5. Absence of pseudoparalysis, axillary nerve palsy

6. Absence of irreparable subscapularis tendon tear

5. Tendon transfers for massive irreparable rotator cuff tears: A review of latissimus dorsi transfer (LDT) and lower trapezius transfer (LTT)

Tendon transfers are another option for massive, irreparable rotator cuff tears. Patients with low-grade rotator cuff arthropathy (Hamada I or II) and a maintained glenohumeral joint with pseudoparalysis are potential candidates. Tendon transfers have been utilized to restore motion, strength, and function via force coupling. From a biomechanical point of view, the transferred tendons are thought to act as humeral head depression and concavity compression (compression of the articulation). They can improve external rotation via a transfer force vector [43]. Latissimus dorsi transfer (LDT) and LTT are both options and can be performed open or with arthroscopic assistance. Indications for LDT and LTT include a relatively young, active patient with a massive irreparable rotator cuff tear, intact deltoid function, without subscapularis deficiency and/or anterior-superior escape of the humerus. The ability to comply with a long rehabilitation protocol is a favorable patient characteristic as well.

LDT was first described by L'Episcopo [44] in the setting of obstetric brachial plexopathy and later adopted by Gerber et al. [45] (**Figures 4** and **5**) for the management of irreparable posterosuperior rotator cuff tears. A level IV study by Gerber et al. studied long-term results of LDT at 10 years follow-up in 46 shoulders. Improvements in flexion, abduction, and external rotation as well as abduction strength were demonstrated. Inferior outcomes were demonstrated in those with subscapularis insufficiency and teres minor atrophy [46]. A recent randomized prospective evaluation of

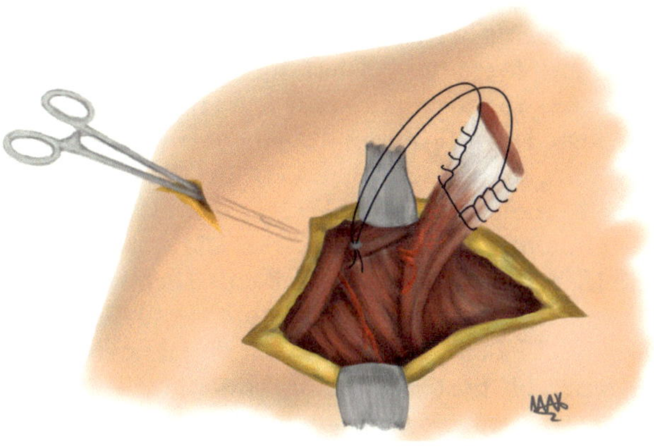

Figure 4.
Through a posterior-based incision, the latisimuss dorsi is harvested from its attachment on the humerus. Nonabsorbable sutures secure the tendon using a locking Krackow technique. The graft is then tunneled through a separate incision deep to deltoid and superficial to infraspinatous.

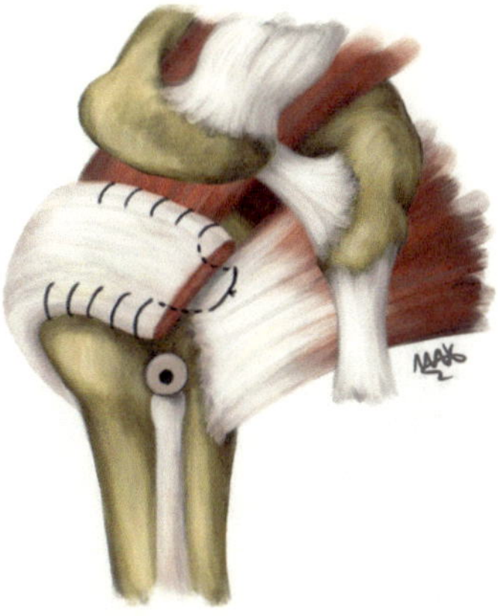

Figure 5.
The lateral edge of the graft is secured on to the greater tuberosity via preferred technique. Remnant supraspinatous can be attached to the medial border of the graft and the distal edge of the graft is secured to upper border of subscapularis (note: long head of biceps tenodesed).

LDT vs. SCR demonstrated that LDT provides statistically significant improvements in range of motion and patient-reported outcomes, although more favorable outcomes in ASES and constant scores were seen in the SCR group [47]. LDT has also been described as option for treatment of subscapularis deficiency with improved function, pain scores, as well as internal rotation in retrospective case series studies [48, 49].

Compared to LDT, LTT offers a better in-line pull similar to the infraspinatus, and biomechanical studies have shown improved external rotation force compared with LDT [50]. Due to the short length of the tendon of the lower trapezius, a bridging graft is necessary. Achilles tendon allograft and semi-tendinosis autograft have both been described in the literature [51, 52]. In either case, the lower trapezius is isolated and harvested from its insertion on the inferomedial scapular spine. Care should be taken not to violate the neurovascular pedicle, including the spinal accessory nerve and transverse cervical artery, which lie medial to the scapula on the undersurface of the muscle. The graft is tunneled through the infraspinatus fascia and under the deltoid and affixed to the greater tuberosity via bone tunnels or suture anchors. The transfer is tensioned with the arm abducted to 90 and in maximal external rotation [52]. Significant improvements in functional scores and active range of motion have been reported across multiple studies [53, 54]. Elhassan et al. reported on 41 patients with irreparable posterior superior rotator cuff tears treated with arthroscopically assisted LTT. They reported significant improvements in visual analog scale, SSV, and disabilities of the arm, shoulder and hand (DASH) scores in 37 of their patients at a mean follow-up of 14 months. Unlike LDT, subscapularis insufficiency was not correlated to inferior outcomes in LTT [53]. A level III retrospective cross-over study comparing LDT with LTT demonstrated greater active external rotation as well as post-operative ASES score. A maintained acromiohumeral distance and a lower progression of arthritis in LTT also revealed that it might be the preferred tendon transfer option for irreparable posterosuperior rotator cuff tears [55]. Rehabilitation after the tendon transfer procedures typically involves 6 weeks of full immobilization in an externally rotated and abducted position, followed by an additional 6 weeks of limited internal or external rotation to protect the transfer.

Although outcomes are suboptimal compared to primary RTC repair, LDT and LTT can serve as attractive options for younger patients with massive, irreparable rotator cuff tears (**Figure 6**).

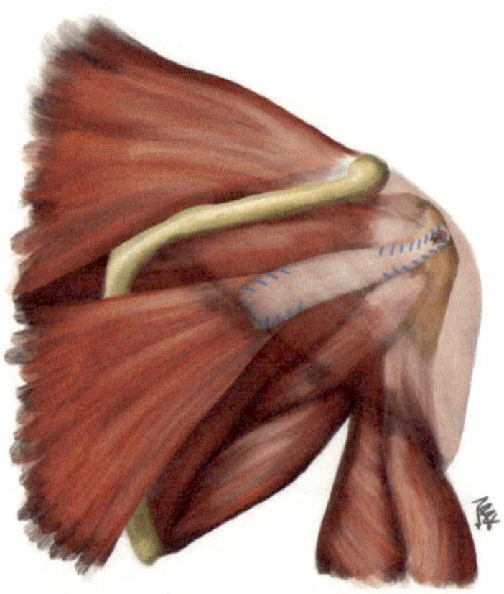

Figure 6.
LTT with utilization of bridging achilles tendon autograft to allow insertion onto greater tuberosity.

6. Anterior cable reconstruction with long head of biceps tendon: A novel technique for rotator cuff repair

The rotator cable is a semi-circular thickening that interweaves with the supraspinatus and infraspinatus tendons. It runs perpendicular to the tendon fibers and blends anteriorly with subscapularis. The analogy of the rotator cable acting as a load-bearing suspension bridge is described by Burkhart et al. [56]. Anatomically, the rotator cable is about 2.59 times thicker than the rotator crescent and provides a stress shielding effect to the thinner tissue of the rotator crescent, where the rotator cuff is inherently prone to tearing [56]. Being a critical structure in biomechanical functioning of the rotator cuff, there have been efforts to address this surgically during the repair of a torn rotator cuff tendon.

ACR with a long head of biceps tendon (LHBT) was described by Park et al. in 2018 [57]. The LHBT is a good graft option for several reasons. It has a proximal attachment on the glenoid, close to the native capsule, and does not require fixation of graft on to the glenoid. The LHBT is often tenotomized, and the proximal stump of tissue is discarded. Thus, it represents a local, expendable, and autologous source of tissue, obviating donor site morbidity as well as foreign body reaction and inflammation associated with nonautologous sources of tissue.

After arthroscopic evaluation of the LHBT, the subacromial space is entered using a standard posterior viewing portal and lateral working portal, and a tuberosity footprint is prepared. A posterolateral viewing portal is made at the posterior edge of a torn tendon in the subacromial space. A triple-loaded medial anchor is then placed at the anterior border of infraspinatus on the cartilage junction. A biceps tenodesis is performed at the site of this anchor. The arm is externally rotated to reduce the strain that may restrict the range of motion. One suture knot is made anterior and one posterior to the tendon and suture remnants after tenodesis as well. A pair of strands that have not been used are then passed through the rotator cuff tendon which are utilized for side-to-side repair over the tenodesis biceps tendon (**Figure 7**). A lateral anchor is then inserted where the anteriorly moved infraspinatus and distal portion of LHBT tendon can lie together. Each of the paired strands is passed through the LHBT and rotator cuff and tied. A biceps tenotomy is then performed (**Figure 7**) [58].

Biomechanically, this has been shown to decrease superior translation of the humeral head and normalize subacromial contact pressures without limiting the range of motion. Clinically, a level III retrospective study of 41 arthroscopic rotator cuff repairs with ACR and 84 without ACR in patients was performed in rotator cable deficient full-thickness supraspinatous tendon tear >2 cm. This demonstrated equivalent VAS, ASES, and ROM but statistically significantly improved acromiohumeral distance and retear rates (4.9% vs. 7.1%) at minimum follow-up of 12 months [58].

Multiple variations of ACR have been described such as a LHBT rerouting procedure [58, 59]. In this procedure, LHBT is mobilized from surrounding soft tissue. A groove is created more laterally on the tuberosity and biceps tenodesis performed in the rerouted position. The rotator cuff repair is completed with the LHBT interposed between the rotator cuff and humeral head (**Figure 7**) [60]. A case series of 80 patients with a large rotator cuff tear and a follow-up of 21 months demonstrated statistically significant improvement in ASES, Korean Shoulder Score, active ROM, and acromiohumeral distance compared with preoperative scores [60].

ACR is an emerging novel technique utilized with good success in a limited number of preliminary studies. There is an increasing level of interest in such techniques,

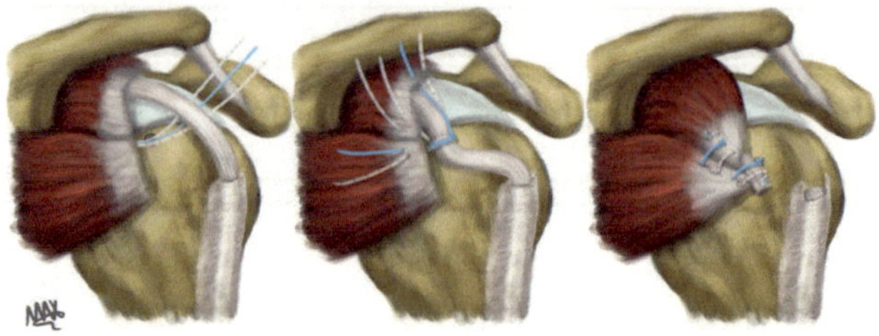

Figure 7.
Schematic depiction of ACR using long head of biceps autograft.

but higher-level comparative studies are lacking and are needed to define the role of ACR in irreparable rotator cuff tears (**Figure** 7).

7. Bursal acromial reconstruction

The evolution of arthroscopic techniques led to the creation of methods such as superior capsule reconstruction, which utilize allografts [61]. However, the SCR is time-consuming, potentially complex, and expensive. This led to the evolution of the BAR, a technique that provides an interposition allograft graft preventing contact between the humerus and acromion [62]. Potential advantage of BAR is lower cost, lower post-operative rehab demands, and anesthesia time compared with techniques such as SCR, tendon transfers, and reverse total shoulder arthroplasty.

Patients are prepared for the surgery by being placed in the beach chair position or the lateral decubitus, ensuring that the acromioclavicular joint (ACJ) is within the surgical field [62]. A bursectomy, minimal acromioplasty, and a lateral clavicle excision is performed with the intention of providing a flat surface for graft insertion and tying around the acromion [62]. The acromial surface area is then measured, and the allograft is trimmed to that measurement. A crossed suture tape configuration with a lasso-loop knot is then created at each corner by passing a high tensile nonabsorbable suture from corner to corner [62]. A suture tape retriever is then placed through the Neviaser portal, and a suture manipulator is placed through the mid-ACJ port [62]. The tape from the posteromedial graft corner is then introduced into a cannula and passed off to the retriever within the Neviaser portal. After insertion of the tape into the anteromedial corner of the graft in the subacromial space, the graft is passed into the waiting tape retriever within the ACJ portal. After all three sutures are inserted, the graft can now be inserted within the subacromial space. After insertion of the graft under the acromion, the three lateral sutures are to be passed via a needle in outside-in-technique [62]. After the passage of all six sutures in the bursa, the corresponding tails are then retrieved for tying [62].

BAR is best indicated for patients with complex rotator cuff tears who are older than 75 years of age and do not show any osteoarthritis [62]. While older

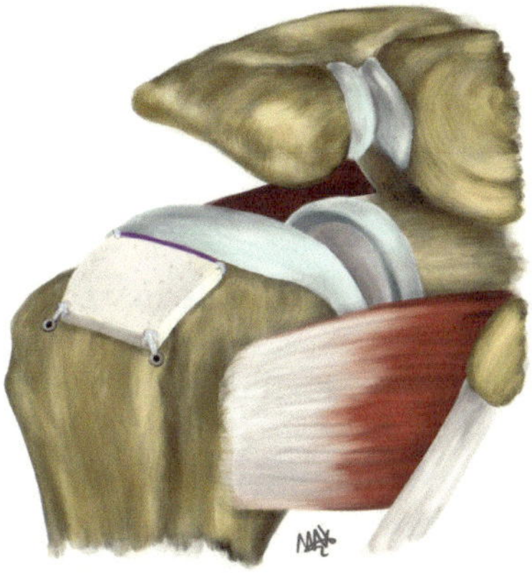

Figure 8.
Arthroscopic view of a dermal allograft affixed to the greater tuberosity.

osteoarthritic patients, or older patients with a torn rotator cuff typically undergo a RSA some can qualify to possibly undergo a BAR [63]. RSA has shown excellent clinical outcomes in patients who undergo the procedures, but not all patients who undergo an RSA may be good candidates [63, 64]. This can include comorbidities or desire to not undergo an arthroplasty [64]. In the case of irreparable rotator cuffs in the elderly, BAR can also be an alternative within those cases. With BAR being a very new procedure, little information on long-term patient outcomes is available. One study, however, released mid-term outcomes for patients undergoing BAR. Patients demonstrated significantly improved Western Ontario Rotator cuff score, and the disabilities of the arm, shoulder, and hand improved, with 92% and 74% of patients meeting clinical differences for the scores respectively (**Figure 8**) [65].

8. Biologic tuberoplasty: A novel option for massive irreparable rotator cuff tears in low-demand patients

For patients with significant comorbidities who are unable to undergo an extensive procedure to treat massive irreparable rotator cuff tears, surgical treatment options are limited. Biologic tuberoplasty is a novel procedure that provides a quicker, bone-sparing option for massive, irreparable rotator cuff tears in low-demand patients. Ideally, patients have little to no glenohumeral joint arthritis [66, 67]. Coverage of tuberosity with an acellular dermal allograft is thought to act as interpositional tissue and prevent bone-on-bone contact between the undersurface of the acromion and the tuberosity, leading to pain relief. The phenomenon of "biologic tuberoplasty" was first described by Mirzayan et al. They noted that patients who had undergone SCR, and had a graft failure, still had equivalent visual analog scale scores and functional outcome scores as patients with intact graft. It was postulated that the residual graft left on the greater tuberosity was preventing bone-on-bone contact with the acromion. In a case series study of 10 patients, there was a significant improvement in ASES, SANE, and VAS scores at a mean follow-up of 21 months with magnetic resonance imaging evidence of healed graft onto the tuberosity in all cases [68]. This novel technique does not, however, restore normal glenohumeral joint kinematics and is intended solely for pain relief. The clinical benefits of this novel technique have yet to be proven with high-level comparative studies. Further comparative data is needed to understand short and long-term outcomes.

Advantages:

1. Lower cost relative to prosthetic replacement.

2. Decreased time under anesthesia for high-risk patients.

3. Avoidance of complications of prosthetic replacement.

4. Low-demand postoperative rehabilitation.

5. Does not increase the difficulty of prosthetic replacement at a later time.

Disadvantages/risks and/or limitations:

1. Cost of dermal allograft.

2. Use of implant, technical risk of foreign body reaction.

3. Does not restore normal glenohumeral joint kinematicsis intended solely as a pain reliever (**Figure 9**).

9. Platelet-rich plasma: An emerging supplementation in rotator cuff repair

The use of platelet-rich product (PRP) supplementation is a particular area of interest in orthopedic surgery. PRP is a biologically active concentrate produced by centrifuging of whole blood. PRP has been utilized in an attempt to improve biologic healing environment as a standalone treatment and adjunct supplementation at the time of rotator cuff repair surgery. Four types of PRP exist depending on preparation: pure platelet-rich plasma (P-PRP), leukocyte- and platelet-rich plasma (L-PRP), pure

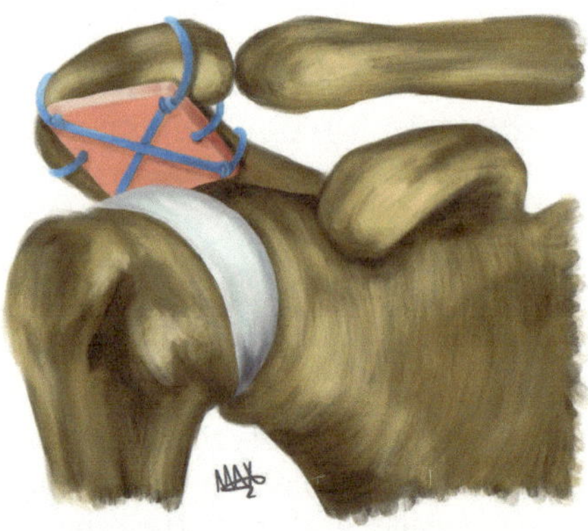

Figure 9.
Schematic of a BAR.

platelet-rich fibrin (P-PRF), and leukocyte- and platelet-rich fibrin (L-PRF) [69]. It contains numerous growth factors important for tissue repair and wound healing such as transforming growth factor B1, platelet-derived growth factor, vascular endothelial growth factor, epithelial growth factor, and insulin-like growth factors [70–72]. There have been extensive research on clinical utility of PRP at time of rotator cuff repair, with mixed results [73, 74]. Recent meta-analysis of randomized controlled trials by Ryan et al. in 2021. This study included 17 level I or II randomized controlled trials comparing 553 patients treated with PRP to 551 control patients with varying size and severity of rotator cuff tears [75]. This study demonstrated favorable results for using PRP in conjunction with rotator cuff repair with lower retear rates. It improved constant scores SST scores, and VAS scores compared to the control group, with P-PRP appearing to be the most effective formulation. Other biologics such as bone marrow aspirate concentrate and stem cells are under investigation; however, clinical data in the setting of rotator cuff repair surgery is lacking.

10. Conclusion

Despite arthroscopic rotator cuff repair being one of the most frequently performed orthopedic procedures, it carries a significant failure rate.

Recent research has focused on addressing both biological and structural concerns of repair, with the emergence of adjuvant repair techniques aimed at improving biology and novel structural techniques developed to augment or replicate the structural properties of rotator cuff. These techniques include biologic patch augmentation, subacromial balloon spacers, tendon transfers, SCR, ACR, BAR, and biologic tuberoplasty.

Further studies are needed to evaluate the efficacy and safety of these emerging techniques. However, the currently available clinical outcomes are encouraging, and these techniques hold great promise in improving the management of rotator cuff tears, especially in the setting of irreparable rotator cuff tears.

Author details

James Young Jin Lee, Mazen Zamzam, Maxwell Li, Alex Martusiewicz, Brett P. Wiater and Jerome Michael Wiater*
Department of Orthopaedic Surgery, Corewell Health William Beaumont University Hospital, Royal Oak, MI, USA

*Address all correspondence to: j.michael.wiater@corewellhealth.org

References

[1] Chakravarty K, Webley M. Shoulder joint movement and its relationship to disability in the elderly. Journal of Rheumatology. 1993;**20**:1359-1361

[2] Largacha M, Parsons IM, Campbell B, Titelman RM, Smith KL, Matsen F. Deficits in shoulder function and general health associated with sixteen common shoulder diagnoses: A study of 2674 patients. Journal of Shoulder and Elbow Surgery. 2006;**15**:30-39

[3] Flatow EL, Soslowsky LJ, Ticker JB, Pawluk RJ, Hepler M, Ark J, et al. Excursion of the rotator cuff under the acromion. Patterns of Subacromial Contact. The American Journal of Sports Medicine. 1994;**22**:779-788

[4] Tempelhof S, Rupp S, Seil R. Age-related prevalence of rotator cuff tears in asymptomatic shoulders. Journal of Shoulder and Elbow Surgery. 1999;**8**:296-299

[5] Chang KV, Hung CY, Han DS, Chen WS, Wang TG, Chien KL. Early versus delayed passive range of motion exercise for arthroscopic rotator cuff repair: A meta-analysis of randomized controlled trials. The American Journal of Sports Medicine. 2015;**43**:1265-1273

[6] Minagawa H, Yamamoto N, Abe H, Fukuda M, Seki N, Kikuchi K, et al. Prevalence of symptomatic and asymptomatic rotator cuff tears in the general population: From mass-screening in one village. Journal of Orthopaedics. 26 Feb 2013;**10**(1):8-12. DOI: 10.1016/j.jor.2013.01.008. PMID: 24403741; PMCID: PMC3768248

[7] Kim YS, Chung SW, Kim JY, Ok JH, Park I, Oh JH. Is early passive motion exercise necessary after arthroscopic rotator cuff repair? The American Journal of Sports Medicine. 2012;**40**:815-821

[8] Keener JD, Galatz LM, Stobbs-Cucchi G, Patton R, Yamaguchi K. Rehabilitation following arthroscopic rotator cuff repair: A prospective randomized trial of immobilization compared with early motion. Journal of Bone and Joint Surgery. American Volume. 2014;**96**:11-19

[9] Tashjian RZ, Hollins AM, Kim HM, Teefey SA, Middleton WD, Steger-May K, et al. Factors affecting healing rates after arthroscopic double-row rotator cuff repair. The American Journal of Sports Medicine. 2010;**38**:2435-2442

[10] Slabaugh MA, Nho SJ, Grumet RC, Wilson JB, Seroyer ST, Frank RM, et al. Does the literature confirm superior clinical results in radiographically healed rotator cuffs after rotator cuff repair? Arthroscopy. 2010;**26**:393-403

[11] Galatz LM, Ball CM, Teefey SA, Middleton WD, Yamaguchi K. The outcome and repair integrity of completely arthroscopically repaired large and massive rotator cuff tears. Journal of Bone and Joint Surgery. American Volume. 2004;**86**:219-224

[12] Ponce BA, Hosemann CD, Raghava P, Tate JP, Sheppard ED, Eberhardt AW. A biomechanical analysis of controllable intraoperative variables affecting the strength of rotator cuff repairs at the suturetendon interface. The American Journal of Sports Medicine. 2013;**41**:2256-2261

[13] Sugaya H, Maeda K, Matsuki K, Moriishi J. Repair integrity and

functional outcome after arthroscopic double-row rotator cuff repair: A prospective outcome study. Journal of Bone and Joint Surgery. American Volume. 2007;**89**(5):953-960

[14] Kim SJ, Kim SH, Lee SK, Seo JW, Chun YM. Arthroscopic repair of massive contracted rotator cuff tears: Aggressive release with anterior and posterior interval slides do not improve cuff healing and integrity. Journal of Bone and Joint Surgery. American Volume. 2013;**95**:1482-1488

[15] Boileau P, Brassart N, Watkinson DJ, Carles M, Hatzidakis AM, Krishnan S. Arthroscopic repair of full-thickness tears of the supraspinatus: Does the tendon really heal? Journal of Bone and Joint Surgery. American Volume. 2005;**87**(6):1229-1240

[16] Cole BJ, McCarty LP III, Kang RW, Alford W, Lewis PB, Hayden JK. Arthroscopic rotator cuff repair: Prospective functional outcome and repair integrity at minimum 2-year follow-up. Journal of Shoulder and Elbow Surgery. 2007;**16**(5):579-585

[17] Ozaki J, Fujimoto S, Masuhara K, Tamai S, Yoshimoto S. Reconstruction of chronic massive rotator cuff tears with synthetic materials. Clinical Orthopaedics and Related Research. Jan 1986;**202**:173-183. PMID: 3955946

[18] Burkhead WZ, Schiffern SC, Krishnan SG. Use of Graft-Jacket as an augmentation for massive rotator cuff tears. Seminars in Arthroplasty. 2007;**18**:11-18

[19] Sclamberg SG, Tibone JE, Itamura JM, Kasraeian S. Six-month magnetic resonance imaging follow-up of large and massive rotator cuff repairs reinforced with porcine small intestinal submucosa. Journal of Shoulder and Elbow Surgery. 2004;**13**:538-541

[20] Iannotti JP, Codsi MJ, Kwon YW, Derwin K, Ciccone J, Brems J. Porcine small intestine submucosa augmentation of surgical repair of chronic two-tendon rotator cuff tears. Journal of Bone & Joint Surgery. 2006;**88-A**(6):1238-1244

[21] Bushnell BD, Connor PM, Harris HW, Ho CP, Trenhaile SW, Abrams JS. Two-year outcomes with a bioinductive collagen implant used in augmentation of arthroscopic repair of full-thickness rotator cuff tears: Final results of a prospective multicenter study. Journal of Shoulder and Elbow Surgery. Dec 2022;**31**(12):2532-2541. DOI: 10.1016/j.jse.2022.05.025. Epub 2022 Jul 1. PMID: 35788057

[22] Avanzi P, Giudici LD, Capone A, et al. Prospective randomized controlled trial for patch augmentation in rotator cuff repair: 24-Month outcomes. Journal of Shoulder and Elbow Surgery. 2019;**28**:1918-1927

[23] Cai YZ, Zhang C, Jin RL, et al. Arthroscopic rotator cuff repair with graft augmentation of 3-dimensional biological collagen for moderate to large tears: A randomized controlled study. The American Journal of Sports Medicine. 2018;**46**:1424-1431

[24] Barber FA, Herbert MA, Boothby MH. Ultimate tensile failure loads of a human dermal allograft rotator cuff augmentation. Arthroscopy. 2008;**24**(1):20-24

[25] Beniker D, McQuillan D, Livesey S, et al. The use of acellular dermal matrix as a scaffold for periosteum replacement. Orthopedics. 2003;**26**(5 Suppl):s591-s596

[26] Adams JE, Zobitz ME, Reach JS Jr, An KN, Steinmann SP. Rotator cuff

repair using an acellular dermal matrix graft: An in vivo study in a canine model. Arthroscopy. 2006;**22**(7):700-709

[27] Barber AF, Burns JP, Deutsch A, Labbé MR, Litchfield RB. A prospective, randomized evaluation of acellular human dermal matrix augmentation for arthroscopic rotator cuff repair. Journal of Arthroscopic & Related Surgery. 2012;**28**(1):8-15. DOI: 10.1016/j.arthro.2011.06.038

[28] Mori D, Kizaki K, Funakoshi N, Yamashita F, Mizuno Y, Shirai T, et al. Irreparable large to massive rotator cuff tears with low-grade fatty degeneration of the infraspinatus tendon: Minimum 7-year follow-up of fascia autograft patch procedure and partial repair. The American Journal of Sports Medicine. 2021;**49**(13):3656-3668. DOI: 10.1177/03635465211043501

[29] Mihata T, Lee TQ, Watanabe C, Fukunishi K, Ohue M, Tsujimura T, et al. Clinical results of arthroscopic superior capsule reconstruction for irreparable rotator cuff tears. Arthroscopy. 2013;**29**(3):459-470

[30] Hirahara AM, Adams CR. Arthroscopic superior capsular reconstruction for treatment of massive irreparable rotator cuff tears. Arthroscopy Techniques. 2015;**4**(6):e637-e641

[31] Noyes MP, Denard PJ. Arthroscopic superior capsular reconstruction: Indications and outcomes. Operative Techniques in Sports Medicine. 2018;**26**(1):29-34

[32] Hartzler RU, Burkhart SS. Superior capsular reconstruction. Orthopaedics. 2017;**40**(5):271-280

[33] Denard PJ, Brady PC, Adams CR, Tokish JM, Burkhart SS. Preliminary results of arthroscopic superior capsule reconstruction with dermal allograft. Arthroscopy. 2018;**34**(1):93-99

[34] Pennington WT, Bartz BA, Pauli JM, Walker CE, Schmidt W. Arthroscopic superior capsular reconstruction with acellular dermal allograft for the treatment of massive irreparable rotator cuff tears: Short-term clinical outcomes and the radiographic parameter of superior capsular distance. Arthroscopy. 2018;**34**(6):1764-1773

[35] Dimock RAC, Malik S, Consigliere P, Imam MA, Narvani AA. Superior capsule reconstruction: What do we know? Archives of Bone and Joint Surgery. 2019;**7**(1):3-11 PMID: 30805409; PMCID: PMC6372269

[36] Parikh N, Martinez DJ, Winer I, Costa L, Dua D, Trueman P. Direct and indirect economic burden associated with rotator cuff tears and repairs in the US. Current Medical Research and Opinion. 2021;**37**(7):1199-1211

[37] Cvetanovich GL, Waterman BR, Verma NN, Romeo AA. Management of the irreparable rotator cuff tear. JAAOS-Journal of the American Academy of Orthopaedic Surgeons. 2019;**27**(24):909-917

[38] Savarese E, Romeo R. New solution for massive, irreparable rotator cuff tears: The subacromial "biodegradable spacer". Arthroscopy Techniques. 2012;**1**(1):e69-e74

[39] Johns WL, Ailaney N, Lacy K, Golladay GJ, Vanderbeck J, Kalore NV. Implantable subacromial balloon spacers in patients with massive irreparable rotator cuff tears: A systematic review of clinical, biomechanical, and financial implications. Arthroscopy, Sports Medicine, and Rehabilitation. 2020;**2**(6):e855-e872

[40] Gervasi E, Maman E, Dekel A, Cautero E. Fluoroscopy-guided biodegradable spacer implantation using local anesthesia: Safety and efficacy study in patients with massive rotator cuff tears. Musculoskeletal Surgery. 2016;**100**(Suppl. 1):19-24. DOI: 10.1007/s12306-016-0433-0

[41] Hazra ROD, Hazra MED, Hanson JA, Millett PJ. The InSpace balloon: Useful augmentation or first-line therapy? Commentary on an article by Nikhil Verma, MD, et al. "InSpace Implant Compared with Partial Repair for the Treatment of Full-Thickness Massive Rotator Cuff Tears. A Multicenter, Single-Blinded, Randomized Controlled Trial". Journal of Bone & Joint Surgery. 2022;**104**(14):e65

[42] Metcalfe A, Parsons H, Parsons N, et al. Subacromial balloon spacer for irreparable rotator cuff tears of the shoulder (START:REACTS): A group-sequential, double-blind, multicentre randomised controlled trial. Lancet. 2022;**399**(10339):1954-1963

[43] Henseler JF, Nagels J, Nelissen RG, de Groot JH. Does the latissimus dorsi tendon transfer for massive rotator cuff tears remain active postoperatively and restore active external rotation? Journal of Shoulder and Elbow Surgery. 2014;**23**:553-560. DOI: 10.1016/j.jse.2013.07.055

[44] L'Episcopo JB. Tendon transplantation in obstetrical paralysis. American Journal of Surgery. 1934;**25**(1):122-125

[45] Gerber C, Vinh TS, Hertel R, et al. Latissimus dorsi transfer for the treatment of massive tears of the rotator cuff. Clinical Orthopaedics and Related Research. 1988;**232**:51-61

[46] Gerber C, Rahm SA, Catanzaro S, et al. Latissimus dorsi tendon transfer for treatment of irreparable posterosuperior rotator cuff tears: Long-term results at a minimum follow-up of ten years. Journal of Bone & Joint Surgery. 2013;**95**(21):1920-1926

[47] Ozturk BY, Ak S, Gultekin O, Baykus A, Kulduk A. Prospective, randomized evaluation of latissimus dorsi transfer and superior capsular reconstruction in massive, irreparable rotator cuff tears. Journal of Shoulder and Elbow Surgery. 2021;**30**(7):1561-1571. DOI: 10.1016/j.jse.2021.01.036 Epub 2021 Mar 4. PMID: 33675971

[48] Kany J, Guinand R, Croutzet P, et al. Arthroscopic-assisted latissimus dorsi transfer for subscapularis deficiency. European Journal of Orthopaedic Surgery and Traumatology. 2016;**26**(3):329-334

[49] Elhassan BT, Wagner ER, Kany J. Latissimus dorsi transfer for irreparable subscapularis tear. Journal of Shoulder and Elbow Surgery. 2020;**29**(10):2128-2134

[50] Reddy A, Gulotta LV, Chen X, et al. Biomechanics of lower trapezius and latissimus dorsi transfers in rotator cuff–deficient shoulders. Journal of Shoulder and Elbow Surgery. 2019;**28**(7):1257-1264

[51] Aibinder WR, Elhassan BT. Arthroscopic lower trapezial transfer for irreparable rotator cuff tears. Operative Techniques in Orthopaedics. 2018;**28**(4):217-225

[52] Elhassan BT, Alentorn-Geli E, Assenmacher AT, et al. Arthroscopic-assisted lower trapezius tendon transfer for massive irreparable posterior-superior rotator cuff tears: Surgical technique. Arthroscopy Techniques. 2016;**5**(5):e981-e988

[53] Elhassan BT, Sanchez-Sotelo J, Wagner ER. Outcome of arthroscopically

assisted lower trapezius transfer to reconstruct massive irreparable posteriorsuperior rotator cuff tears. Journal of Shoulder and Elbow Surgery. 2020;**29**(10):2135-2142

[54] Stone MA, Kane LT, Ho JC, et al. Short-term outcomes of lower trapezius tendon transfer with Achilles allograft for irreparable posterosuperior rotator cuff tears. Arthroscopy, Sports Medicine, and Rehabilitation. 2021;**3**(1):e23-e29

[55] Baek C, Lee D, Kim J. Lattisimus dorsi transfer vs. lower trapezius transfer for posterosuperior irreparable rotator cuff tears. Journal of Shoulder and Elbow Surgery. 2022;**31**:1810-1822

[56] Burkhart SS, Esch JC, Jolson RS. The rotator crescent and rotator cable: An anatomic description of the shoulder's "suspension bridge". Arthroscopy. 1993;**9**(6):611-616. DOI: 10.1016/s0749-8063(05)80496-7 Erratum in: Arthroscopy 1994 Apr;10(2):239. PMID: 8305096

[57] Park SR, Sun DH, Kim J, et al. Is augmentation with the long head of the biceps tendon helpful in arthroscopic treatment of irreparable rotator cuff tears? Journal of Shoulder and Elbow Surgery. 2018;**27**:1969-1977

[58] Shin S, Kim I, Park I, Lee S, Kim M. Anterior cable reconstruction using the biceps tendon in retracted anterior L-shaped rotator cuff tears. Arthroscopy Techniques. 2021;**10**(1):e55-e60

[59] Seo J, Kwak K, Park B, Yoo J. Anterior cable reconstruction using the proximal biceps tendon for reinforcement of arthroscopic rotator cuff repair prevent retear and increase acromiohumeral distance. Journal of Orthopaedics. 2021;**23**:246-249

[60] Kim J, Lee H, Park T, Lee J, Kim Y. Preliminary outcomes of arthroscopic biceps rerouting for the treatment of large to massive rotator cuff tears. Journal of Shoulder and Elbow Surgery. 2021;**30**:1384-1392

[61] Tokish JM, Beicker C. Superior capsule reconstruction technique using an acellular dermal allograft. Arthroscopy Techniques. 2015;**4**:e833-e839

[62] Ravenscroft M, Barnes MW, Muench LN, Mazzocca AD, Berthold DP. Bursal acromial reconstruction (BAR) using an acellular dermal allograft as a surgical solution for the treatment of massive irreparable rotator cuff tears. Arthroscopy Techniques. 2021;**10**(3):e877-e885. DOI: 10.1016/j.eats.2020.11.002. PMID: 33738228; PMCID: PMC7953327

[63] Mulieri P, Dunning P, Klein S, Pupello D, Frankle M. Reverse shoulder arthroplasty for the treatment of irreparable rotator cuff tear without glenohumeral arthritis. Journal of Bone and Joint Surgery. American Volume. 2010;**92**:2544-2556

[64] Petrillo S, Longo UG, Papalia R, Denaro V. Reverse shoulder arthroplasty for massive irreparable rotator cuff tears and cuff tear arthropathy: A systematic review. Musculoskeletal Surgery. 2017;**101**:105-112

[65] Awad MA, Sparavalo S, Ma J, King JP, Wong I. Interposition graft bridging reconstruction of irreparable rotator cuff tears using acellular dermal matrix: Medium-term results. Arthroscopy: The Journal of Arthroscopic & Related Surgery. 2022;**38**(3):692-698

[66] Mirzayan R, Bouz G. Biologic tuberoplasty with an acellular dermal allograft for massive rotator cuff

tears. Arthroscopy Techniques. 2021;**10**:e1743-e1749. DOI: 10.1016/j.eats.2021.03.016

[67] Griffin JW, Runzo D, Bonner KF. Arthroscopic biologic interpositional tuberosity graft for the treatment of irreparable rotator cuff tears. Arthroscopy Techniques. 2021;**10**:e1729-e1735. DOI: 10.1016/j.eats.2021.03.024

[68] Mirzayan R. Preliminary outcomes of arthroscopic biologic tuberoplasty in the treatment of massive irreparable rotator cuff tears. Cureus. 2023;**15**(1):e34402. DOI: 10.7759/cureus.34402

[69] Ehrenfest, David M. Dohan, et al. Classification of platelet concentrates (Platelet-Rich Plasma-PRP, Platelet-Rich Fibrin-PRF) for topical and infiltrative use in orthopedic and sports medicine: Current consensus, clinical implications and perspectives. Muscles, Ligaments and Tendons Journal 2014;**4**(1):3

[70] Arnoczky SP, Delos D, Rodeo SA. What is platelet-rich plasma? Operative Techniques in Sports Medicine. 2011;**19**(142-148):23

[71] Sanchez M, Azofra J, Aizpurua B, Andıa I, Anitua E. Use of autologous plasma rich in growth factors in arthroscopic surgery. Cuadernos de Artroscopia. 2003;**10**(12-19):24

[72] Anitua E, Sanchez M, Nurden AT, et al. Autologous fibrin matrices: A potential source of biological mediators that modulate tendon cell activities. Journal of Biomedical Materials Research. 2006;**77**:285-293

[73] Hurley ET, Lim Fat D, Moran CJ, Mullett H. The efficacy of platelet-rich plasma and platelet-rich fibrin in arthroscopic rotator cuff repair: A meta-analysis of randomized controlled trials. The American Journal of Sports Medicine. 2019;**47**:753-761

[74] Warth RJ, Dornan GJ, James EW, Horan MP, Millett PJ. Clinical and structural outcomes after arthroscopic repair of full-thickness rotator cuff tears with and without platelet-rich product supplementation: A meta-analysis and meta-regression. Arthroscopy. 2015;**31**:306-320

[75] Ryan J, Imbergamo C, Sudah S, Kirchner G, Greenberg P, Monica J, et al. Platelet-rich product supplementation in rotator cuff repair reduces retear rates and improves clinical outcomes: A meta-analysis of randomized controlled trials. Arthroscopy. 2021;**37**(8):2608-2624. DOI: 10.1016/j.arthro.2021.03.010

Chapter 3

Arthroscopic Treatment for Massive Cuff Tears

Petru Razvan Melinte

Abstract

In the current literature, several definitions are provided for massive cuff tears. At the same time, a massive cuff tear can be reparable or irreparable. As a consequence, certain criteria need to be defined to address this issue of reparability—quality of tendon, status of muscle atrophy, bone of greater tuberosity, status of glenohumeral joint, and last but not least the clinical criterion, that is the functionality of shoulder. Several arthroscopic treatment options are described — from simple biceps tenotomy, partial reconstruction techniques with or without biologic augmentation, and superior capsule reconstruction to other rather new tools such as balloon spacer implantation.

Keywords: massive tear, cuff, arthroscopic, shoulder, treatment

1. Introduction

What is a massive rotator cuff tear? The definition is somehow inconsistent. Cofield [1] defined a massive cuff tear as a tear with a width larger than 5 cm; Gerber [2] defined an MCT intraoperatively as a tear that after extensive debridement appears to affect two or more tendons; other authors [3] take into consideration an exposure of the humeral head wider than 3 cm, which usually has a surface of more than 9 cm. On the other hand, Hamada and Fukuda looked at X-rays in patients with MCT and described the elevation of the humeral head in the absence of glenohumeral arthritis, and they proposed their well-known classification. However, if we analyze these definitions for MCT, they take into consideration the size but make no indication regarding reparability; therefore, an MCT is not necessarily an irreparable tear. Hamada and Fukuda radiologic classification indicates that when the tear is chronic and its chronicity leads to humeral head elevation, then it is generally accepted that the tear should be considered irreparable. Surgeons should understand this important distinction, as an MCT can be reparable when it is acute or most likely irreparable in a chronic situation.

So, the next thing that needs to done is to define what is irreparable; irreparable can be considered as being both unfixable and unhealable. Unfixable is the inability to physically repair the tendon back to bone after expensive releases. Irreparable may be also unhealable, as described by Gerber [2], as any repair that is achieved but that will most likely be followed by failure, such as the need for reoperation due to retear,

IntechOpen

poor postoperative motion or strength, or poor outcome [4]. The Gold standard of irreparability is intraoperative inability to repair after extensive releases.

Nevertheless, most of the times, it is difficult preoperatively to decide if an RC tear is irreparable; surgeons must also take into consideration intraoperative findings. In general, arguments of irreparability include advanced fatty infiltration according to Goutallier classification (Goutallier grade 3 or more), decreased acromiohumeral distance (less than 6 mm), dramatic decrease of tendon length, and poor-quality tendon tissue.

Pascal Boileau [5] looked at the problem from a different perspective and gave us 7 good reasons not to repair an RCT: no tendon, due to resorbtion; no rotator cuff muscle, due to atrophy, fatty infiltration; no good bone – greater tuberosity osteoporosis seen especially in women; no good joint – glenohumeral osteoarthritis; static superior and anterior humeral head subluxation; dynamic humeral head subluxation, due to pseudoparalysis; and previous surgery – destroyed anterior deltoid, low grade infection.

Patients with a massive cuff tear usually complain about shoulder pain and decrease of function, which is often declared as decrease of active anterior elevation and/or active external rotation; the symptoms may be singular or in combination. Generally, three questions need to be asked: is this shoulder functional or not? is the muscle balance preserved; second—is the long head of biceps present, as a painful shoulder can be caused by a long head of biceps subluxation; and third — in which plane is the shoulder unbalanced—vertical plane, horizontal plane, or both. Answering these questions may help us choose the right treatment tailored to the patients' symptoms and the type of shoulder muscle imbalance. The management of irreparable rotator cuff tears can be achieved by both surgical and nonsurgical methods that can address both functional and non-functional shoulders. Certainly, we must consider non-operative treatment for the right patient—usually nonsurgical treatment consists of: medication such as anti-inflammatory drugs, injection of corticosteroids substances inside subacromial space, and physical therapy.

While non-functional shoulder may benefit from tendon transfers and/or reverse shoulder arthroplasty, for functional shoulders, there are several surgical options for repairing massive rotator cuff tears. Despite the rapidly increasing numbers of reverse shoulder arthroplasties, alternative options are available [6–18]; among those, we mention biceps tenotomy or tenodesis, arthroscopic debridement, partial repair, complete repair, augmentation of repair with different types of patches, superior capsular reconstruction, and muscle tendon transfer [19]. Recently, superior capsular deficiency can be treated by the use of various autografts/allograft; respected shoulder surgeons present several surgical techniques such as: rerouting the long head of biceps tendon, use of long head of biceps tendon as an autograft, use of semitendinosus as an allograft, or simpler methods — subacromial spacers [20]. In the literature [19, 21], there is a lack of consensus and lack of guidelines on the appropriate indications for specific surgical treatment options, although, recent work from [20, 22] present an agreement on treatment of massive irreparable rotator cuff tears by the Neer Circle of the American Shoulder and Elbow Surgeons [20, 22].

To improve the success rates of operative results, there are several factors to be considered according to [19, 23] who proposed that some specific aspects should be met in order to achieve the best clinical results: subacromial decompression should be performed thoroughly; integrity of the deltoid muscle fibers origin should be preserved; torn tendons should be adequately mobilized, and interval slide should be done whenever necessary; tendons should be repaired down to bone; postoperative rehabilitation is a must. In addition, Yoon [24] proposed two essential requirements: the repaired rotator cuff should be able to sustain early tension during the initial healing stage, and one must obtain a certain biological environment that favors the healing ability of the repair site—that is, the bone-tendon junction [19]. Thus, surgical treatment performed must ensure decompression and debridement of the subacromial space and considerable strength in the repaired area; in this way, the repaired rotator cuff will be able to stabilize the glenohumeral joint; at the same time, we emphasize once more that providing a good biological environment will sustain a maximum healing capacity, allowing for safe mobilization [19, 23].

2. Debridement and biceps Tenotomy

Arthroscopic debridement was traditionally applied to massive rotator cuff tears in old patients with comorbidities and low functional expectations [19, 21, 25]. Early results presented clinical benefits such as decreased symptoms and improved range of motion. Berth et al. [19, 26] published several studies proving that debridement alone is associated with temporary benefits; debridement alone did not improve shoulder strength [19, 27]. Consequently, as new arthroscopic repair techniques emerged, debridement has become less popular.

Biceps tendon lesions are an important source of shoulder pain and often accompany massive rotator cuff tears. Greenspoon et al. [19, 21] confirmed that shoulder pain and dysfunction are reduced after biceps tenotomy or tenodesis, inducing good satisfaction in patients [19]; however, the natural history of rotator cuff tears is not influenced by biceps procedures alone [19]. In addition, some studies [19] showed no significant clinical improvements after arthroscopic debridement and biceps tenotomy when compared to arthroscopic debridement alone [19, 21].

Another systematic review study [4] demonstrates that arthroscopic debridement procedures are followed by good midterm to long-term patient outcomes; all 16 included studies presented significant clinical improvement in pain and range of motion. Thus, arthroscopic debridement is presented as a safe and reproducible surgical option with a low risk of complication (4.1%) [4]. The included studies presented in [4] seem to underline that pain relief has a greater importance than improvements of shoulder function in patients older than 65 years that underwent debridement.

Walch et al. [28] reported that patients with MCT treated nonoperatively declared pain relief after spontaneous long head of the biceps ruptures [19, 28]. They compared these findings to the results after arthroscopic biceps tenotomy in the same category of patients; similar improvements in pain and range of motion were observed. But these studies involving biceps showed decreases in the acromiohumeral distance, which seems logical if one takes into consideration the depressor effect of the long head of the biceps onto the humeral head [19, 29, 30]. Interestingly, patients still declared reduced pain and slightly better outcomes despite associated superior humeral head elevation [19, 29, 30]. Walch [28] also mentioned that fatty infiltration had negative prognostic effect on function and X-ray progression of arthritis.

Boileau [31] presented 72 irreparable cuff tears treated with tenotomy and debridement showing 78% satisfied patients; according to his observations, teres minor atrophy worsens prognosis, and he considered pseudoparalysis and severe cuff arthropathy as contraindication.

3. Rotator cuff repair

When compared to other surgical techniques, arthroscopic repair seems to lead to the best results, at least from a clinical point of view [32, 33]. Nevertheless, even when the tear is repaired anatomically, it may have a low chance of healing. There are some factors that are related to tendon, such as the chronicity of the tear, the quality of the muscle, and the pattern and size of the tear that were proved to be associated to a low healing rate [34–36]. The healing of rotator cuff is additionally negatively influenced by other factors related to the age of patients and their comorbidities like smoking, hyperlipidemia, and diabetes [32, 37]. In conclusion, if we take into account the patient and its tendon-related factors, the ideal tear for repair is in a patient that still has a good joint space, with an X-ray that can be classified as Hamada 1 or 2, while clinical examination reveals preserved range of motion [32, 38, 39]. Massive tears in patients that present with pseudoparalysis that occurred in the last 6 months should be arthroscopically repaired as studies have proved that pseudoparalysis can be reversed [32, 39]. But, neglected pseudoparalysis or pseudoparalysis that appeared as a complication of a repair is less likely to recover into a good functional shoulder [32].

As emphasized above, it is generally agreed among surgeons that a complete repair of a massive cuff tear should tempt to completely restore the anatomic insertion of tendon to footprint, but in some patients, this goal cannot be achieved due to shortening of torn tendons, as muscles contract and retract quickly [40]. In such cases, a partial repair, although incomplete and not anatomic, can be tried [40]. Arthroscopic partial repair is advised in patients that are young and have a preserved structure of muscle with quite a low fatty infiltration that can be quantified using the MRI-based Fuchs classification [41]. In order to improve the functional results, these types of procedures can be performed together with a tendon transfer; depending on the location of the irreparable tear, the tendon used for transfer may be: latissimus dorsi or lower trapezius muscle fibers in case of posterosuperior tears; pectoralis major or sometimes latissimus dorsi in anterosuperior tears [40]. Arthroscopic partial repair and/or tendon transfer for MCT was proved to lead to satisfactory outcomes as claimed by quite a number of clinical studies [26, 40, 42–51].

Recently, a systematic review of the literature [40] was published; it inquired internet databases about studies dealing with arthroscopic repair of MCT; 55 studies have been identified, and 11 clinical studies were considered eligible, comprising 643 patients. Muscle strength was found to be significantly improved in all studies, while the functional range of motion was noted in the majority of cases [40]. Apparently, even a partial repair allows the shoulder to get balance and become less painful and more mobile [40, 52]. All these accomplishments are possible apparently with a low reoperation and complication rate [40]. Revision surgery had rarely to be performed because in case of repair failure, it was rather uncommon for the patient to complain about persistent pain [40]. So, as an intermediate conclusion, arthroscopic partial repair is a safe salvage solution [40]. Postoperative MRI or ultrasound found the retear rate to be about 50% [40]. The actual value of partial repair is challenged by this quite elevated risk of failure; much controversy is raised by the continuous improvement in symptoms and functionality even when the structural integrity of the repaired cuff is altered [40]. Lubiatowski [53] claims that clinical outcomes are not influenced by the preserved integrity of the repaired cuff [40, 53]. This finding might be explained by the increase of muscle strength after lavage, debridement, and synovectomy; consequently, there is less pain induced by muscle activity, so the status of repair would not matter anymore [26, 40, 54]. If the surgeon adds a decompression of suprascapular nerve, then the clinical outcome will significantly improve and will not be affected by the structural integrity of the repaired cuff [40, 55].

Nevertheless, there are some drawbacks to the previously mentioned studies [26, 40, 42–51] as the number of patients surveyed was quite small, the follow-up was widely variable, and long-term follow-up was not reported in any of the studies cited [40, 42–51]. With that being said, the value of arthroscopic partial repair technique needs to be proved by new studies dealing with the long-term patient outcomes [40]. Other negative aspects are that some papers dealt with heterogeneous populations characterized by different muscle structural anomalies such as fatty infiltration and by different sizes and numbers of tendon lesions [40, 42–51]. Finally, when we review the literature, even the type of the surgical procedure was not exactly the same as surgeons performed arthroscopic partial repair differently; some used a medialization of footprint in order to reduce tension of the repaired cuff [40, 56]; others were more conservative and applied margin convergence technique described by Burkhart [40, 57].

As an intermediate conclusion, we may say that arthroscopic partial repair might be an effective solution for contracted massive cuff tear, where an anatomic and complete repair cannot be achieved. The benefits are that it may improve strength and may improve the outcome of operation while restoring the muscle force couples, but it dramatically increases recovery if you treat it like a standard cuff repair; in old age populations where there is a low chance of healing, the question that is raised is: are you creating more morbidity? And last but not least, as mentioned before [40, 42–51], the quality of the available literature is low or at most moderate.

4. Mechanical and biological augmentation of rotator cuff repair

In order to promote and improve healing after partial/complete repair of massive cuff tears, various patch augmentation devices have been developed; according to the structure and origin of the graft, they may be synthetic extracellular matrix scaffolds, xenograft, and allograft [19, 58]. There are no clear recommendations for implanting scaffolds in rotator cuff surgery, but augmentation through the use of extracellular matrix patches is being investigated [19].

Scaffold augmentation is promoted because it can support mechanically the repair especially during the sensitive early phase of healing; other researchers state that they can also supply a network to accommodate the migrated cells that are mandatory for the healing process at the tendon-to-bone interface [19]. To this extent, synthetic scaffolds ensure structural and mechanical support and maintain the stability of the repair, gaining time until the tissue heals; they do not influence directly the biological environment at the repair [19, 59–62].

The use of scaffolds derived from human dermis led to the improvement of shoulder scores and a better structural integrity of the repair, when implanted as an augment (85% in augmentation group vs. 40% in control group) [19, 61–65]; histologic samples from the repair site with augmentation showed no inflammation, infection, or calcifications at 3 months after surgery. But these scaffolds used for augmentation have a lower elasticity when compared to tendons, and therefore, theoretically, the repaired construct may have a higher tear rate [19, 60–62].

Extracellular matrix xenografts still pose the problem of immunogenicity despite adequate cell removal during the rigorous graft preparation process [60]; there are recommendations against these augmentation scaffolds, because in a high percentage of patients, important inflammatory responses have been signaled [19, 66, 67]. Other studies, like those conducted by Throckmorton and Gerlinger [19, 58], present favorable outcomes with dermal-origin scaffolds. Throckmorton and Gerlinger [19, 58] studies have also presented statistical information showing a decrease of clinical symptoms and an increase in function, strength, and shoulder scores.

Another graft option could be synthetic polymer implants that have no immunologic risk [19]. Synthetic extracellular matrix scaffolds proved to significantly increase the functionality of the repaired RCT [19, 58, 68]. A comparative study investigating patients with cuff surgery augmented by xenograft or synthetic graft noted retearing rates at 1-year follow-up of 51% and 17%, respectively, when related to 41% in patients with no augmentation [19, 60, 69].

Advanced research on the biology of healing of the rotator cuff tears, deep to the cellular level, even in augmented repaired cuff tears opened the path to new direct therapies [19]. Cellular growth factors applied at the repair site in animal studies induced neovascularization and cell proliferation [19]. However, the mechanical quality of the repair and tendon resistance to load did not improve according to these studies [19]. In another article, Cheung et al. [70, 71] stated that growth factors may enhance tendon-to-bone healing, *in vivo*.

The application of orthobiologics during arthroscopic rotator cuff repair has gained increasing clinical interest in the past decade, despite clear evidence studies; they are supposed to enhance tendon healing and improve clinical outcomes [72].

Platelet-rich plasma (PRP) is an autologous blood-derived fluid that contains growth factors; some of them are considered to be crucial in bone-to-tendon healing [19, 71]. The growth factors in PRP include an insulin-like growth factor-1, platelet-derived growth factor, vascular endothelial growth factor, and transforming growth factor-b [19, 73]. Theoretically, PRP at the repair site should promote healing, but there is controversy over its role because of contradictory results reported in the literature [60]. Many shoulder surgeons advocate that there is not enough evidence for the benefit of PRP biologic augmentation in any rotator cuff repair [19, 74–77].

Ryan et al. [78] conducted a comprehensive systematic review and meta-analysis to determine the influence of different types of platelet-rich plasma as an augmentation procedure to rotator cuff repair; 17 studies were investigated, and the influence of leukocyte and platelet-rich plasma, leukocyte and platelet-rich fibrin, pure platelet-rich plasma (P-PRP), and pure platelet-rich fibrin was observed; the conclusion was that all types of PRP significantly reduce retear rate, especially when P-PRP is used [78].

In another study, Feltri et al. [79] looked at 36 randomized controlled trials and concluded that the augmentation with PRP reduces the retear rate but has no benefits on clinical outcomes; the same study [79] pointed out that PRP in patients treated conservatively failed to present any clear advantage.

Besides PRP, bone marrow aspirate concentrate (BMAC) has rapidly spread as an alternative biological therapy to augment tendon-to-bone healing.

Schoch et al. [72] investigated the effect of bone marrow aspirate concentrate (BMAC) and platelet-rich plasma augmentation on the rate of revision rotator cuff repair; the study included a total of 760 patients who underwent biological augmentation during rotator cuff repair — 646 patients with PRP and 114 patients with BMAC. They concluded that the application of BMAC led to a significant decrease in the rate of revision surgery, but there was no apparent effect of PRP.

But, Cole et al. [80] in a prospective randomized trial found out that BMAC-augmented arthroscopic repair of isolated supraspinatus tendon tears largely fails to improve failure rates and clinical outcomes when compared with simple arthroscopic repair.

Muench et al. [81] developed and published an arthroscopic technique biologically augmented with PRP, autologous subacromial bursa tissue, platelet-poor plasma (PPP), concentrated bone marrow aspirate, and bovine thrombin as stabilizer; a recent case series of patients treated with a very similar technique showed improvement in functional outcomes and quite a substantial clinical benefit [82].

Stem cells have multiple differentiation potentials, which stimulate tendon remodeling and increase biomechanical strength [83]. Additionally, stem cell-derived extracellular vesicles (EVs) can increase collagen synthesis while inhibiting inflammation and adhesion formation by carrying regulatory proteins and microRNAs [83]. Taking all that into account and reading all the literature available, stem cell-based therapy in rotator cuff repair seems to be the future, although basic clinical research is definitely required [83].

5. Superior capsular reconstruction

The superior capsule of glenohumeral joint spans from the superior labrum to the greater tuberosity of humerus; it covers the footprint of the supraspinatus tendon, and from a biomechanical point of view, it acts like a static stabilizer for the glenohumeral joint [19, 20, 84–87].

Biomechanically, superior capsule reconstruction (SCR) can restore and thus regain balance of the force couples necessary for shoulder function [19, 20, 84]. Superior capsule is a static stabilizer that reduces the glenohumeral, allowing muscles like the deltoid and pectoralis major to function in proper conditions [19, 20, 84, 85, 87]. Superior capsular reconstruction is indicated in patients with irreparable tear of posterior superior cuff but with minimal or no glenohumeral arthritis (Hamada stage 1 and 2) and functional deltoid and trapezius; force couples should be balanced in the transverse plane, that is, intact teres minor and intact or reparable subscapularis, in other words—Type C and D according to Collin classification [34].

Mihata [85] observed the superior translation of humeral head, secondary increased acromiohumeral pressure, and associated low joint compression force while studying the biomechanical properties of glenohumeral joints with irreparable supraspinatus tears [85, 88, 89]. As an operative solution, he described the reconstruction of superior capsule (SCR) using a fascia lata as an autograft [85, 88, 89]. He fixed the fascia lata autograft to the scapular neck and the opposite side to the greater tuberosity; the interposed autograft would prevent the superior migration of the humeral head [19, 85, 88–91].

Mihata [85] published excellent clinical results even in mid-term follow-up studies. The American Shoulder and Elbow Surgeons score increased from 29 preoperatively to 83 and 92 postoperatively after one year and five years, respectively; forward elevation increased from 85° preoperatively to 138° and 151° postoperatively after one year and five years, respectively; acromiohumeral distance also improved (preoperative—3.4 mm; one year postoperatively—9.1 mm; five years after surgery—8.1 mm) [19, 20, 91].

Harvesting fascia lata was linked to donor site morbidity and longer surgery times, so as a consequence, allogenic dermal allografts have been introduced. These allografts have been proven to act biomechanically like fascia lata to restore the humeral head position after a massive rotator cuff tear [19, 20, 92]. Burkhart et al. [19, 20, 93] used allograft reconstruction of superior capsule, and the published results are promising; in their series; they reported improvements of clinical outcome, quantified by American Shoulder and Elbow Surgeons and visual analog scale scores that increased from 45.6 to 85.8 and 5.26 to 0.96, respectively, at one year postoperatively [19, 20, 93].

Despite the relatively high costs of SCR with allograft (cost of dermal allograft and a large number of anchors used for appropriate fixation), SCR does not restore the active function of the supraspinatus muscle; therefore, some would consider these observations as drawbacks of the procedure. However, the technique still represents a viable treatment option in young and active patients who would not favor shoulder replacement [19, 20].

6. Other arthroscopic techniques for superior stabilization of humeral head

Recently, the long head of biceps tendon has been utilized in numerous surgical techniques to reconstruct the superior capsule [12, 13, 16, 22, 86, 94, 95]. These techniques are classified into techniques that reroute the tendon and techniques that use the tendon as a graft [19, 20]. All of these procedures require an intact long head of biceps tendon and seize the opportunity to harvest a locally available and viable autograft. In shoulders with intact long head of biceps tendon and intact glenohumeral cartilage, the use of biceps tendon for superior stabilization of the humeral head led to good clinical outcomes [19, 20].

Kim [17] published a technique that uses the long head of biceps tendon to perform *in situ* reconstruction of the superior capsule. In this technique, intraarticular biceps tenotomy is performed keeping the labral attachment intact; then, the freed end of tendon is fixed at the level of greater tuberosity; thus, biceps tendon pushes down the humeral head, reducing superior humeral head migration [19, 20].

Han [14] used seven fresh frozen shoulders to analyze from a biomechanical point of view this rerouting procedure; the results were promising, showing a stable shoulder as this rerouting technique successfully centers the humeral head into the glenoid cavity, thus reducing subacromial contact pressure and allowing for a functional range of motion [14, 19, 20]. To further support this technique, Sang-Yup Han [87] conducted biomechanical experimental studies on eight cadaveric shoulders and investigated the effects of biceps tendon rerouting with and without associated rotator cuff repair; the results reported a lower translation of humeral head, a more centered head with secondary reduced subacromial pressure, and no negative influence on the rotational range of motion [19, 20, 94]. When used in combination to arthroscopic cuff repair, this rerouting technique resulted in low retear rates and good clinical outcomes [15, 20, 96, 97]. However, data for an isolated biceps rerouting for massive irreparable rotator cuff tears are not available yet [15, 20, 96, 97].

Tang and Zhao [16, 19, 20] introduced a similar technique called arthroscopic *dynamic* rerouting; they created a new bicipital groove lateral to the native bicipital grove; the tendon is not attached at the level of greater tuberosity. Until now, clinical or biomechanical data have not been published [19, 20].

In a systematic review comparing superior capsular reconstruction techniques using long head of biceps tendon, Kitridis [93] arrived to the conclusion that these new biceps rerouting techniques were easy, time-efficient, and cost-effective [19, 20].

Denard [13] introduced another surgical technique that uses the biceps tendon in a box configuration; he supported his proposal with a biomechanical study on eight cadaveric shoulders. Apparently, in patients with massive rotator cuff tears, the technique did not restore the translation to previous range, although it decreased superior migration of the humeral head [13, 19, 20]. Clinical results for this technique have not been published yet [20]. Kim [17] proposed a variant of this technique that takes long head of biceps tendon with both its intraarticular and extraarticular parts and reconstructs the superior capsule; he referred to it as the Snake/Triple Bundle technique [17, 20]; the biceps tendon was sutured with tape, and an open subpectoral tenodesis was performed as an additional procedure. No clinical data have been reported yet [20].

Milano [98] used a semitendinosus tendon autograft and presented a surgical technique for superior capsular reconstruction. The semitendinosus tendon is harvested and debrided; then, it is armed with non-absorbable sutures; the graft is attached with anchors at the superior part of glenoid neck; the surgeon can create a box shape, V-shape, or reverse V-shape, depending on the graft length, and then attach it to the previously decorticated greater tuberosity [19, 20, 98, 99].

Bader and Garcia in 2020 [100] proposed the pivot superior capsular reconstruction fixation technique; it also uses a semitendinosus autograft that is shuttled through a hole in the scapular neck and then fixed in the greater tuberosity, preferably with an interference screw [19, 20, 100]. In 2021, Berthold [101] published a biomechanical cadaver study, investigating the best biceps and other graft rerouting surgical techniques; the results suggested that the V- shape and box-shape configurations significantly decreased superior humeral head migration and decreased deltoid cumulative forces [20, 101].

7. Biodegradable balloon

The subacromial spacer was approved by the US-FDA (Food and Drug Administration), for the treatment of MIRCTs, in 2021.

In 2012, in their studies, Romeo and Savarese [102] proposed the use of InSpace balloon, due to its simple and easy applicability technique [20, 102]. Consisting of poly-l-lactide-co-ε-caprolactone, the pre-shaped InSpace spacer has an adsorption time of 1 year (12 months) [20, 102–105]. As a surgical technique, the first step is the usual method of debridement and bursectomy, followed by positioning the biodegradable-type spacer through the lateral portal. Afterwards, a 0.9% saline solution is inserted, with the help of a Luer-Lock syringe, using the application system [20, 102]. The balloon size is proportional to the inserted volume of saline solution. Balloon sizing depends either on the tear and shoulder morphology or on the arthroscopic probe measurements, so their size varies, from small—40 × 50 mm, to medium—50 × 60 mm and large—60 × 70 mm [20, 102].

The long-term as well as mid-term outcomes and efficiency have been debated, due to the fact that the balloon is biodegradable within 1 year (12 months) [20, 98]. In a prospective study conducted by Familiari [103], 51 patients (mean age 63 – range 50–78 years old) were observed during a mean period of 36 months (24–56 months) [20, 103]. The results of Familiari's prospective research showed improvement of Constant Score (CS) from 27 ± 7.4 up to 77 ± 15 ($P \leq 0.01$). Furthermore, good to excellent scores were described in 46 patients, while five patients experienced unsatisfactory outcomes [20, 103]. Currently, in the existing literature, for the treatment options in massive irreparable rotator cuff tears, there are no comparative studies between other methods and InSpace Balloon technique [20].

8. Bursal acromial resurfacing

Based on the concept of subacromial spacer, in his study, Ravenscroft [106] proposed a special surgical technique, known as bursal acromial resurfacing (BAR). This procedure consists of an allograft—dermal-type, acellular—regarded as an option for irreparable rotator cuff tears [20].

Elderly patients (70 years old or over) presenting minimal or even no osteoarthritic evidences should benefit from this type of surgery. With the purpose of, on one hand, reducing the pain and, on the other hand, decreasing down to the minimum humeral head-acromion contact, as authors stated [20, 106], this surgical procedure should mix both grafts' longevity, together with balloon simplicity. So far, no further evidence, such as clinical results, have been presented [20, 106].

9. Arthroscopic biologic inter-positional tuberosity graft

The greater tuberosity is a rare place for the dermal allografts to fail [107, 108]; instead, they usually fail within the graft's mid-substance or at the glenoid level [20, 107, 108]. The clinical and imagistic study described by Mirazayan [109] showed that even failed dermal-type allograft superior capsular reconstruction relieves pain and improves functional outcomes [20, 109]; this observation could be explained by the so called "Biologic Tuberoplasty Effect" [20, 110].

As it is placed between the greater tuberosity and acromion, the graft is regarded as an interposition, biologic spacer, having a role in restricting the painful contact between these structures. Clinical outcomes for this type of procedures still require more studies and are not conclusive yet.

Author details

Petru Razvan Melinte
University of Medicine and Pharmacy from Craiova, Romania

*Address all correspondence to: razvan.melinte@gmail.com

References

[1] Cofield RH. Rotator cuff disease of the shoulder. The Journal of Bone and Joint Surgery. American Volume. 1985;**67**:974-979

[2] Gerber C, Fuchs B, Hodler J. The results of repair of massive tears of the rotator cuff. The Journal of Bone and Joint Surgery. American Volume. 2000;**82**:505-515

[3] Nobuhara K, Hata Y, Komai M. Surgical procedure and results of repair of massive tears of the rotator cuff. Clinical Orthopaedics and Related Research. Jul 1994;(304):54-59. PMID: 8020234

[4] Soderlund M, Boren M, O'Reilly A, San JA, Mahlys JM. Arthroscopic debridment for management of massive, irreparable rotator cuff tears: A systematic review of outcomes. JSES Reviews, Reports and Techniques. 2022;**2**:1-7

[5] Boileau P, Andreani O, Schramm M, Baba M, Barret H, Chelli M. The effect of tendon delamination on rotator cuff healing. The American Journal of Sports Medicine. 2019;**47**(5):1074-1081. DOI: 10.1177/0363546519835491

[6] Marigi EM, Johnson QJ, Dholakia R, Borah BJ, Sanchez-Sotelo J, Sperling JW. Cost comparison and complication profiles of superior capsular reconstruction, lower trapezius transfer, and reverse shoulder arthroplasty for irreparable rotator cuff tears. Journal of Shoulder and Elbow Surgery. 2022;**31**:847-854. DOI: 10.1016/j.jse.2021.08.027

[7] Gerber C. Latissimus dorsi transfer for the treatment of irreparable tears of the rotator cuff. Clinical Orthopaedics and Related Research. 1992;**275**:152-160. Available from: https://pubmed.ncbi.nlm.nih.gov/1735206/

[8] Waltenspül M, Jochum B, Filli L, Ernstbrunner L, Wieser K, Meyer D, et al. Mid-term results of arthroscopically assisted latissimus dorsi transfer for irreparable posterosuperior rotator cuff tears. Journal of Shoulder and Elbow Surgery. 2021;**30**:e676-e688. DOI: 10.1016/j.jse.2021.03.149

[9] Elhassan BT, Sanchez-Sotelo J, Wagner ER. Outcome of arthroscopically assisted lower trapezius transfer to reconstruct massive irreparable posterior-superior rotator cuff tears. Journal of Shoulder and Elbow Surgery. 2020;**29**:2135-2142. DOI: 10.1016/j.jse.2020.02.018

[10] Gerber C, Rahm SA, Catanzaro S, Farshad M, Moor BK. Latissimus dorsi tendon transfer for treatment of irreparable posterosuperior rotator cuff tears: Long-term results at a minimum follow-up of ten years. Journal of Bone and Joint SurgeryAmerican Volume. 2013;**95**:1920-1926. DOI: 10.2106/JBJS.M.00122

[11] Samuelsen BT, Wagner ER, Houdek MT, Elhassan BT, Sánchez-Sotelo J, Cofield R, et al. Primary reverse shoulder arthroplasty in patients aged 65 years or younger. Journal of Shoulder and Elbow Surgery. 2017;**26**:e13-e17. DOI: 10.1016/j.jse.2016.05.026

[12] Tang D, Jang Y, Park J, On M. Arthroscopic superior capsular reconstruction with biceps autograft: Snake technique. Arthroscopy Techniques. 2019;**8**:e1085-e1092

[13] Denard PJ, Chae S, Chalmers C, Choi JH, McGarry MH, Adamson G,

et al. Biceps box configuration for superior capsule reconstruction of the glenohumeral joint decreases superior translation but not to native levels in a biomechanical study. Arthroscopy, Sports Medicine, and Rehabilitation. 2021;**3**:e343-e350

[14] Han F, Kong CH, Hasan MY, Ramruttun AK, Kumar VP. Superior capsular reconstruction for irreparable supraspinatus tendon tears using the long head of biceps: A biomechanical study on cadavers. Orthopaedics & Traumatology, Surgery & Research. 2019;**105**:257-263. DOI: 10.1016/j.otsr.2018.10.023

[15] Rhee SM, Youn SM, Park JH, Rhee YG. Biceps rerouting for semirigid large-to-massive rotator cuff tears. Arthroscopy. 2021;**37**:2769-2779. DOI: 10.1016/j.arthro.2021.04.008

[16] Tang J, Zhao J. Dynamic biceps rerouting for irreparable posterior-superior rotator cuff tear. Arthroscopy Techniques. 2020;**9**:e1709-e1714. DOI: 10.1016/j.eats.2020.07.014

[17] Kim YS, Lee HJ, Park I, Sung GY, Kim DJ, Kim JH. Arthroscopic in situ superior capsular reconstruction using the long head of the biceps tendon. Arthroscopy Techniques. 2018;**7**:e97-e103. DOI: 10.1016/j.eats.2017.08.058

[18] Colbath G, Murray A, Siatkowski S, Pate T, Krussig M, Pill S, et al. Autograft long head biceps tendon can be used as a scaffold for biologically augmenting rotator cuff repairs. Arthroscopy. 2022;**38**:38-48. DOI: 10.1016/j.arthro.2021.05.064

[19] Joseph Y. Rho, Yong suk Kwon, Sungwook Choi. Current concepts and recent trends in arthroscopic treatment of large to massive rotator cuff tears: A review, Clinics in Shoulder and Elbow. 2019;**22**(1):50-57. DOI: 10.5397/cise.2019.22.1.50

[20] Dey Hazra ME, Dey Hazra R, Hanson JA, Ganokroj P, Vopat ML, Rutledge JC, et al. Treatment options for massive irreparable rotator cuff tears: A review of arthroscopic surgical options. EFORT Open Reviews. 2023;**8**(1):35-44. Retrieved Aug 25, 2023, from. DOI: 10.1530/EOR-22-0015

[21] Greenspoon JA, Petri M, Warth RJ, Millett PJ. Massive rotator cuff tears: Pathomechanics, current treatment options, and clinical outcomes. Journal of Shoulder and Elbow Surgery. 2015;**24**(9):1493-1505. DOI: 10.1016/j.jse.2015.04.005

[22] Pierre P, Millett PJ, Abboud JA, Cordasco FA, Cuff DJ, Dines DM, et al. Consensus statement on the treatment of massive irreparable rotator cuff tears: A Delphi approach by the Neer circle of the American shoulder and elbow surgeons. Journal of Shoulder and Elbow Surgery. 2021;**30**:1977-1989. DOI: 10.1016/j.jse.2021.05.012

[23] Azar FM, Canale ST, Beaty JH. Campbell's Operative Orthopaedics. 13th ed. Amsterdam: Elsevier; 2016. pp. 2298-2345

[24] Yoon JP. Patch augmentation for massive rotator cuff tears. Clinics in Shoulder and Elbow. 2017;**20**(2):105-112. DOI: 10.5397/cise.2017.20.2.105

[25] Gerber C, Wirth SH, Farshad M. Treatment options for massive rotator cuff tears. Journal of Shoulder and Elbow Surgery. 2011;**20**(2 Suppl):S20-S29. DOI: 10.1016/j.jse.2010.11.028

[26] Berth A, Neumann W, Awiszus F, Pap G. Massive rotator cuff tears: Functional outcome after debridement or arthroscopic partial repair. Journal

of Orthopaedics and Traumatology. 2010;**11**(1):13-20. DOI: 10.1007/s10195-010-0084-0

[27] Burkhart SS. Arthroscopic treatment of massive rotator cuff tears. Clinical Orthopaedics and Related Research. 2001;**390**:107-118

[28] Walch G, Edwards TB, Boulahia A, Nové-Josserand L, Neyton L, Szabo I. Arthroscopic tenotomy of the long head of the biceps in the treatment of rotator cuff tears: Clinical and radiographic results of 307 cases. Journal of Shoulder and Elbow Surgery. 2005;**14**:238-246

[29] Klinger HM, Steckel H, Ernstberger T, Baums MH. Arthroscopic débridement of massive rotator cuff tears: Negative prognostic factors. Archives of Orthopaedic and Trauma Surgery. 2005;**125**:261-266

[30] Slim K, Nini E, Forestier D, Kwiatkowski F, Panis Y, Chipponi J. Methodological index for non-randomized studies (minors): Development and validation of a new instrument. ANZ Journal of Surgery. 2003;**73**:712-716

[31] Boileau P, Baqué F, Valerio L, Ahrens P, Chuinard C, Trojani C. Isolated arthroscopic biceps tenotomy or tenodesis improves symptoms in patients with massive irreparable rotator cuff tears. The Journal of Bone & Joint Surgery. 2007;**89**(4):747-757

[32] Ardebol J, Hwang S, Horinek JL, Menendez ME, Pak T, Denard PJ. A step-by-step approach to arthroscopic repair of massive rotator Cuff tears. Arthroscopy Techniques. 2023;**12**(3):e377-e382, ISSN 2212-6287. DOI: 10.1016/j.eats.2022.11.019

[33] Thorsness R, Romeo A. Massive rotator cuff tears: Trends in surgical management. Orthopedics. 2016;**39**:145-151

[34] Collin P, Matsumura N, Lädermann A, Denard PJ, Walch G. Relationship between massive chronic rotator cuff tear pattern and loss of active shoulder range of motion. Journal of Shoulder and Elbow Surgery. 2014;**23**:1195-1202

[35] Abtahi AM, Granger EK, Tashjian RZ. Factors affecting healing after arthroscopic rotator cuff repair. World Journal of Orthopedics. 2015;**6**:211-220

[36] Schanda JE, Eigenschink M, Laky B. Rotator cuff delamination is associated with increased tendon retraction and higher fatty muscle infiltration: A comparative study on arthroscopy and magnetic resonance imaging. Arthroscopy. 2022;**38**:2131-2141.e1

[37] Jensen AR, Taylor AJ, Sanchez-Sotelo J. Factors influencing the reparability and healing rates of rotator cuff tears. Current Reviews in Musculoskeletal Medicine. 2020;**13**:572-583

[38] di Benedetto P, Mancuso F, Tosolini L, Buttironi MM, Beltrame A, Causero A. Treatment options for massive rotator cuff tears: A narrative review. Acta Biomed. 2021;**92**:e2021026

[39] Denard PJ, Lädermann A, Brady PC. Pseudoparalysis from a massive rotator cuff tear is reliably reversed with an arthroscopic rotator cuff repair in patients without preoperative glenohumeral arthritis. The American Journal of Sports Medicine. 2015;**43**:2373-2378

[40] Malahias MA, Kostretzis L, Chronopoulos E, et al. Arthroscopic partial repair for massive rotator cuff

tears: Does it work? A systematic review. Sports Medicine - Open. 2019;**5**:13

[41] Fuchs B, Weishaupt D, Zanetti M, Hodler J, Gerber C. Fatty degeneration of the muscles of the rotator cuff: Assessment by computed tomography versus magnetic resonance imaging. Journal of Shoulder and Elbow Surgery. 1999;**8**:599-605

[42] Cuff DJ, Pupello DR, Santoni BG. Partial rotator cuff repair and biceps tenotomy for the treatment of patients with massive cuff tears and retained overhead elevation: Midterm outcomes with a minimum 5 years of follow-up. Journal of Shoulder and Elbow Surgery. 2016;**25**(11):1803-1809

[43] Franceschi F, Papalia R, Vasta S, Leonardi F, Maffulli N, Denaro V. Surgical management of irreparable rotator cuff tears. Knee Surgery, Sports Traumatology, Arthroscopy. 2015;**23**(2):494-501

[44] Godenèche A, Freychet B, Lanzetti RM, Clechet J, Carrillon Y, Saffarini M. Should massive rotator cuff tears be reconstructed even when only partially repairable? Knee Surgery, Sports Traumatology, Arthroscopy. 2017;**25**(7):2164-2173

[45] Heuberer PR, Kölblinger R, Buchleitner S, et al. Arthroscopic management of massive rotator cuff tears: An evaluation of debridement, complete, and partial repair with and without force couple restoration. Knee Surgery, Sports Traumatology, Arthroscopy. 2016;**24**(12):3828-3837

[46] Holtby R, Razmjou H. Relationship between clinical and surgical findings and reparability of large and massive rotator cuff tears: A longitudinal study. BMC Musculoskeletal Disorders. 2014;**15**:180

[47] Iagulli ND, Field LD, Hobgood ER, Ramsey JR, Savoie FH 3rd. Comparison of partial versus complete arthroscopic repair of massive rotator cuff tears. The American Journal of Sports Medicine. 2012;**40**(5):1022-1026

[48] Kim SJ, Lee IS, Kim SH, Lee WY, Chun YM. Arthroscopic partial repair of irreparable large to massive rotator cuff tears. Arthroscopy. 2012;**28**(6):761-768

[49] Mori D, Funakoshi N, Yamashita F. Arthroscopic surgery of irreparable large or massive rotator cuff tears with low-grade fatty degeneration of the infraspinatus: Patch autograft procedure versus partial repair procedure. Arthroscopy. 2013;**29**(12):1911-1921

[50] Paribelli G, Boschi S, Randelli P, Compagnoni R, Leonardi F, Cassarino AM. Clinical outcome of latissimus dorsi tendon transfer and partial cuff repair in irreparable postero-superior rotator cuff tear. Musculoskeletal Surgery. 2015;**99**(2):127-132

[51] Shon MS, Koh KH, Lim TK, et al. Arthroscopic partial repair of irreparable rotator cuff tears: Preoperative factors associated with outcome deterioration over 2 years. The American Journal of Sports Medicine. 2015;**43**(8):1965-1975

[52] Burkhart SS, Nottage WM, Ogilvie-Harris DJ, et al. Partial repair of irreparable rotator cuff tears. Arthroscopy. 1994;**10**:363-370

[53] Lubiatowski P, Kaczmarek P, Dzianach M, et al. Clinical and biomechanical performance of patients with failed rotator cuff repair. International Orthopaedics. 2013;**37**(12):2395-2401

[54] Mallon WJ, Wilson RJ, Basamania CJ. The association of suprascapular

neuropathy with massive rotator cuff tears: A preliminary report. Journal of Shoulder and Elbow Surgery. 2006;**15**:395-398

[55] Itoi E, Minagawa H, Sato T, et al. Isokinetic strength after tears of the supraspinatus tendon. Journal of Bone and Joint Surgery. British Volume (London). 1997;**79**:77-82

[56] Lee KW, Moon KH, Ma CH, Lee GS, Yang DS, Choy WS. Clinical and radiologic outcomes after medializing and not medializing rotator cuff tendon attachment site on chronic retracted rotator cuff tears. Arthroscopy. Aug 2018;**34**(8):2298-2307. DOI: 10.1016/j.arthro.2018.03.015. PMID: 29804954

[57] Burkhart SS, Athanasiou KA, Wirth MA. Margin convergence: A method of reducing strain in massive rotator cuff tears. Arthroscopy. 1996;**12**(3):335-338

[58] Throckmorton TQ, Gerlinger TL. Instructional course lectures Rosemont (IL). American Academy of Orthopaedic Surgeons. 2016;**65**:93-108

[59] Gerber C, Wirth SH, Farshad M. Treatment options for massive rotator cuff tears. Journal of Shoulder and Elbow Surgery. 2011;**20**(2 Suppl):S20-S29. DOI: 10.1016/j.jse.2010.11.028

[60] Parvizi J, Huddleston JI. Instructional course lectures Rosemont (IL). American Academy of Orthopaedic Surgeons. 2018;**67**:129-142

[61] Wong I, Burns J, Snyder S. Arthroscopic GraftJacket repair of rotator cuff tears. Journal of Shoulder and Elbow Surgery. 2010;**19**(2 Suppl):104-109. DOI: 10.1016/j.jse.2009.12.017

[62] Gilot GJ, Alvarez-Pinzon AM, Barcksdale L, Westerdahl D, Krill M, Peck E. Outcome of large to massive rotator cuff tears repaired with and without extracellular matrix augmentation: A prospective comparative study. Arthroscopy. 2015;**31**(8):1459-1465. DOI: 10.1016/j.arthro.2015.02.032

[63] Barber FA, Burns JP, Deutsch A, Labbé MR, Litchfield RB. A prospective, randomized evaluation of acellular human dermal matrix augmentation for arthroscopic rotator cuff repair. Arthroscopy. 2012;**28**(1):8-15. DOI: 10.1016/j.arthro.2011.06.038

[64] Denard PJ, Jiwani AZ, Lädermann A, Burkhart SS. Long-term outcome of arthroscopic massive rotator cuff repair: The importance of double-row fixation. Arthroscopy. 2012;**28**:909-915. DOI: 10.1016/j.arthro.2011.12.007

[65] Vaishnav S, Millett PJ. Arthroscopic rotator cuff repair: Scientific rationale, surgical technique, and early clinical and functional results of a knotless self-reinforcing double-row rotator cuff repair system. Journal of Shoulder and Elbow Surgery. 2010;**19**(2 Suppl):83-90. DOI: 10.1016/j.jse.2009.12.012

[66] Walton JR, Bowman NK, Khatib Y, Linklater J, Murrell GA. Restore orthobiologic implant: Not recommended for augmentation of rotator cuff repairs. The Journal of Bone and Joint Surgery. American Volume. 2007;**89**(4):786-791

[67] James KS, Cornwell KC, Greenburg AG. Extracellular matrix bioscaffolds for orthopaedic applications. The Journal of Bone and Joint Surgery. American Volume. 2010;**92**(5):1316-1317 author reply 1317-8

[68] Lederman ES, Toth AP, Nicholson GP, et al. A prospective, multicenter study to evaluate clinical and radiographic outcomes in primary rotator

cuff repair reinforced with a xenograft dermal matrix. Journal of Shoulder and Elbow Surgery. 2016;**25**(12):1961-1970. DOI: 10.1016/j.jse.2016.02.029

[69] Ciampi P, Scotti C, Nonis A, et al. The benefit of synthetic versus biological patch augmentation in the repair of posterosuperior massive rotator cuff tears: A 3-year followup study. The American Journal of Sports Medicine. 2014;**42**(5):1169-1175. DOI: 10.1177/0363546514525592

[70] Cheung EV, Silverio L, Sperling JW. Strategies in biologic augmentation of rotator cuff repair: A review. Clinical Orthopaedics and Related Research. 2010;**468**(6):1476-1484. DOI: 10.1007/s11999-010-1323-7

[71] Boswell SG, Cole BJ, Sundman EA, Karas V, Fortier LA. Platelet-rich plasma: A milieu of bioactive factors. Arthroscopy. 2012;**28**(3):429-439. DOI: 10.1016/j.arthro.2011.10.018

[72] Schoch BS, Werner BC, Shapiro SA, Camp CL, Chalmers PN, Cancienne JM. Effect of bone marrow aspirate concentrate and platelet-rich plasma augmentation on the rate of revision rotator cuff repair. Orthopaedic Journal of Sports Medicine. 2022;**10**(11):23259671221127004. DOI: 10.1177/23259671221127004. PMID: 36353396; PMCID: PMC9638537

[73] Kobayashi M, Itoi E, Minagawa H, et al. Expression of growth factors in the early phase of supraspinatus tendon healing in rabbits. Journal of Shoulder and Elbow Surgery. 2006;**15**(3):371-377. DOI: 10.1016/j.jse.2005.09.003

[74] Jo CH, Shin JS, Lee YG, et al. Platelet-rich plasma for arthroscopic repair of large to massive rotator cuff tears: A randomized, single-blind, parallel-group trial. The American Journal of Sports Medicine. 2013;**41**(10):2240-2248. DOI: 10.1177/0363546513497925

[75] Gumina S, Campagna V, Ferrazza G, et al. Use of plateletleukocyte membrane in arthroscopic repair of large rotator cuff tears: A prospective randomized study. The Journal of Bone and Joint Surgery. American Volume. 2012;**94**(15):1345-1352. DOI: 10.2106/JBJS.K.00394

[76] Holtby R, Christakis M, Maman E, et al. Impact of plateletrich plasma on arthroscopic repair of small- to mediumsized rotator cuff tears: A randomized controlled trial. Orthopaedic Journal of Sports Medicine. 2016;**4**(9):2325967116665595. DOI: 10.1177/2325967116665595

[77] Chahal J, Van Thiel GS, Mall N, et al. The role of platelet-rich plasma in arthroscopic rotator cuff repair: A systematic review with quantitative synthesis. Arthroscopy. 2012;**28**(11):1718-1727. DOI: 10.1016/j.arthro.2012.03.007

[78] Ryan J, Imbergamo C, Sudah S, Kirchner G, Greenberg P, Monica J, Gatt C. Platelet-rich product supplementation in rotator cuff repair reduces retear rates and improves clinical outcomes: A meta-analysis of randomized controlled trials. Arthroscopy. 2021;**37**(8):2608-2624. DOI: 10.1016/j.arthro.2021.03.010. Epub 2021 Mar 17. PMID: 33744318; PMCID: PMC8349828

[79] Feltri P, Gonalba GC, Boffa A, et al. Platelet-rich plasma does not improve clinical results in patients with rotator cuff disorders but reduces the retear rate. A systematic review and meta-analysis. Knee Surgery, Sports Traumatology, Arthroscopy. 2023;**31**:1940-1952. DOI: 10.1007/s00167-022-07223-9

[80] Cole BJ, Kaiser JT, Wagner KR, Sivasundaram L, Otte RS, Tauro TM,

White GM, Ralls ML, Yanke AB, Forsythe B, Romeo AA, Verma NN. Prospective randomized trial of biologic augmentation with bone marrow aspirate concentrate in patients undergoing arthroscopic rotator Cuff repair. The American Journal of Sports Medicine 2023;**51**(5):1234-1242. DOI: 10.1177/03635465231154601. Epub 2023 Feb 22. PMID: 36811557

[81] Muench LN, Uyeki CL, Mancini MR, Berthold DP, McCarthy MB, Mazzocca AD. Arthroscopic Rotator Cuff Repair Augmented with Autologous Subacromial Bursa Tissue, Concentrated Bone Marrow Aspirate, Platelet-Rich Plasma, Platelet-Poor Plasma, and Bovine Thrombin. Arthroscopy Techniques. 2021;**10**(9):e2053-e2059, ISSN 2212-6287. DOI: 10.1016/j.eats.2021.05.008

[82] Muench LN, Kia C, Berthold DP, Uyeki C, Otto A, Cote MP, et al. Preliminary clinical outcomes following biologic augmentation of arthroscopic rotator cuff repair using subacromial bursa, concentrated bone marrow aspirate, and platelet-rich plasma. Arthroscopy, Sports Medicine, and Rehabilitation. 2020;**2**(6):e803-e813, ISSN 2666-061X. DOI: 10.1016/j.asmr.2020.07.019

[83] Wang HN, Rong X, Yang LM, Hua WZ, Ni GX. Advances in stem cell therapies for rotator cuff injuries. Frontiers in Bioengineering and Biotechnology. 2022;**10**:866195. DOI: 10.3389/fbioe.2022.866195. PMID: 35694228; PMCID: PMC9174670

[84] Petri M, Greenspoon JA, Millett PJ. Arthroscopic superior capsule reconstruction for irreparable rotator cuff tears. Arthroscopy Techniques. 2015;**4**(6):e751-e755. DOI: 10.1016/j.eats.2015.07.018

[85] Mihata T, McGarry MH, Kahn T, Goldberg I, Neo M, Lee TQ. Biomechanical effect of thickness and tension of fascia Lata graft on glenohumeral stability for superior capsule reconstruction in irreparable supraspinatus tears. Arthroscopy. 2016;**32**:418-426. DOI: 10.1016/j.arthro.2015.08.024

[86] Kitridis D, Yiannakopoulos C, Sinopidis C, Givissis P, Galanis N. Superior capsular reconstruction of the shoulder using the long head of the biceps tendon: A systematic review of surgical techniques and clinical outcomes. Medicina. 2021;**57**:1-12. DOI: 10.3390/medicina57030229

[87] Tokish JM, Beicker C. Superior capsule reconstruction technique using an acellular dermal allograft. Arthroscopy Techniques. 2015;**4**(6):e833-e839. DOI: 10.1016/j.eats.2015.08.005

[88] Mihata T, McGarry MH, Kahn T, Goldberg I, Neo M, Lee TQ. Biomechanical role of capsular continuity in superior capsule reconstruction for irreparable tears of the supraspinatus tendon. American Journal of Sports Medicine. 2016;**44**:1423-1430. DOI: 10.1177/0363546516631751

[89] Mihata T, McGarry MH, Kahn T, Goldberg I, Neo M, Lee TQ. Biomechanical effects of acromioplasty on superior capsule reconstruction for irreparable supraspinatus tendon tears. American Journal of Sports Medicine. 2016;**44**:191-197. DOI: 10.1177/0363546515608652

[90] Greenspoon JA, Petri M, Warth RJ, Millett PJ. Massive rotator cuff tears: Pathomechanics, current treatment options, and clinical outcomes. Journal of Shoulder and Elbow Surgery. 2015;**24**:1493-1505. DOI: 10.1016/j.jse.2015.04.005

[91] Mihata T, Lee TQ, Hasegawa A, Fukunishi K, Kawakami T, Fujisawa Y, et al. Five-year follow-up of arthroscopic superior capsule reconstruction for irreparable rotator cuff tears. The Journal of Bone and Joint Surgery. American Volume. 2019;**101**:1921-1930. DOI: 10.2106/JBJS.19.00135

[92] Lacheta L, Brady A, Rosenberg SI, Dekker TJ, Kashyap R, Zandiyeh P, et al. Superior capsule reconstruction with a –thick dermal allograft partially restores glenohumeral stability in massive posterosuperior rotator cuff deficiency: A dynamic robotic shoulder model. American Journal of Sports Medicine. 2021;**49**:2056-2063. DOI: 10.1177/03635465211013364

[93] Burkhart SS, Denard PJ, Adams CR, Brady PC, Hartzler RU. Arthroscopic superior capsular reconstruction for massive irreparable rotator cuff repair. Arthroscopy Techniques. 2016;**5**(6):e1407-e1418. DOI: 10.1016/j.eats.2016.08.024

[94] Han SY, Lee TQ, Wright DJ, Park IJ, Mauro M, McGarry MH, et al. Effect of biceps rerouting technique to restore glenohumeral joint stability for large irreparable rotator cuff tears: A cadaveric biomechanical study. Journal of Shoulder and Elbow Surgery. 2020;**29**:1425-1434. DOI: 10.1016/j.jse.2019.11.015

[95] Sachinis NP, Papagiannopoulos S, Sarris I, Papadopoulos P. Outcomes of arthroscopic nerve release in patients treated for large or massive rotator cuff tears and associated suprascapular neuropathy: A prospective, randomized, double-blinded clinical trial. American Journal of Sports Medicine. 2021;**49**:2301-2308. DOI: 10.1177/03635465211021834), 10.1177/03635465211021834)

[96] Llinás PJ, Bailie DS, Sanchez DA, Chica J, Londono JF, Herrera GA. Partial superior capsular reconstruction to augment arthroscopic repair of massive rotator cuff tears using autogenous biceps tendon: Effect on retear rate. American Journal of Sports Medicine. 2022;**50**:3064-3072. DOI: 10.1177/03635465221112659

[97] Chiang CH, Shaw L, Chih WH, Yeh ML, Ting HH, Lin CH, et al. Modified superior capsule reconstruction using the long head of the biceps tendon as reinforcement to rotator cuff repair lowers retear rate in large to massive reparable rotator cuff tears. Arthroscopy. 2021;**37**:2420-2431. DOI: 10.1016/j.arthro.2021.04.003

[98] Milano G, Saccomanno MF, Colosio A, Adriani M, Galli S, Scaini A, et al. Arthroscopic superior capsule reconstruction with doubled autologous semitendinosus tendon graft. Arthroscopy Techniques. 2020;**9**:e1665-e1672. DOI: 10.1016/j.eats.2020.07.009

[99] Rosales-Varo AP, Zafra M, García-Espona MA, Flores-Ruiz MA, Roda O. Superior capsular reconstruction of irreparable rotator cuff tear using autologous hamstring graft. Revista Española de Cirugía Ortopédica y Traumatología. 2019;**63**:1-6. DOI: 10.1016/j.recot.2018.08.004

[100] Bader DAL, Garcia JC. Pivot superior capsular reconstruction of the shoulder. Arthroscopy Techniques. 2020;**9**:e697-e701. DOI: 10.1016/j.eats.2020.01.026

[101] Berthold DP, Muench LN, Dyrna F, Scheiderer B, Obopilwe E, Cote MP, et al. Comparison of different fixation techniques of the long head of the biceps tendon in superior capsule reconstruction for

irreparable posterosuperior rotator cuff tears: A dynamic biomechanical evaluation. American Journal of Sports Medicine. 2021;**49**:305-313. DOI: 10.1177/0363546520981559

[102] Savarese E, Romeo R. New solution for massive, irreparable rotator cuff tears: The subacromial "biodegradable spacer". Arthroscopy Techniques. 2012;**1**:e69-e74. DOI: 10.1016/j.eats.2012.02.002

[103] Familiari F, Nayar SK, Russo R, De Gori M, Ranuccio F, Mastroianni V, et al. Subacromial balloon spacer for massive, irreparable rotator cuff tears is associated with improved shoulder function and high patient satisfaction. Arthroscopy. 2021;**37**:480-486. DOI: 10.1016/j.arthro.2020.09.048

[104] Piekaar RSM, Bouman ICE, van Kampen PM, van Eijk F, Huijsmans PE. The subacromial balloon spacer for massive irreparable rotator cuff tears: Approximately 3 years of prospective follow-up. Musculoskeletal Surgery. 2020;**104**:207-214. DOI: 10.1007/s12306-019-00614-1

[105] Guevara BG. Editorial commentary: Balloons for rotator cuff tears: A viable treatment or just a bunch of hot air? Arthroscopy. 2021;**37**:487-488. DOI: 10.1016/j.arthro.2020.11.018

[106] Ravenscroft M, Barnes MW, Muench LN, Mazzocca AD, Berthold DP. Bursal acromial reconstruction (BAR) using an acellular dermal allograft as a surgical solution for the treatment of massive irreparable rotator cuff tears. Arthroscopy Techniques. 2021;**10**:e877-e885. DOI: 10.1016/j.eats.2020.11.002

[107] Lacheta L, Horan MP, Schairer WW, Goldenberg BT, Dornan GJ, Pogorzelski J, et al. Clinical and imaging outcomes after arthroscopic superior capsule reconstruction with human dermal allograft for irreparable posterosuperior rotator cuff tears: A minimum 2-year follow-up. Arthroscopy. 2020;**36**:1011-1019. DOI: 10.1016/j.arthro.2019.12.024

[108] Mihata T, Lee TQ, Watanabe C, Fukunishi K, Ohue M, Tsujimura T, Kinoshita M. Clinical results of arthroscopic superior capsule reconstruction for irreparable rotator cuff tears. Arthroscopy. 2013;**29**:459-470. DOI: 10.1016/j.arthro.2012.10.022

[109] Mirzayan R, Bouz G. Biologic tuberoplasty with an acellular dermal allograft for massive rotator cuff tears. Arthroscopy Techniques. 2021;**10**:e1743-e1749. DOI: 10.1016/j.eats.2021.03.016

[110] Griffin JW, Runzo D, Bonner KF. Arthroscopic biologic interpositional tuberosity graft for the treatment of irreparable rotator cuff tears. Arthroscopy Techniques. 2021;**10**:e1729-e1735. DOI: 10.1016/j.eats.2021.03.024

Section 2

Knee

Chapter 4

Graft Choice in Anterior Cruciate Ligament Reconstruction

Adrian Todor

Abstract

Anterior cruciate ligament (ACL) reconstruction is one of the most frequent surgical procedures performed by the sports medicine orthopedic surgeon. Many factors can influence the final outcome of the procedure, and the graft used is one of them. Over the years, the surgical technique has evolved and has been refined, including tunnel placement, graft fixation, and graft choice. For the latter, the main options available to the surgeon are autografts, which include patellar tendon, hamstring tendons, and quadriceps tendon autografts, allografts, and synthetic grafts. The ideal option for graft material, if there is one, is still to be determined. All graft options have advantages and disadvantages. Usually, the operating surgeon's preference or recommendation will determine the graft to be used, as such it is very important to have a complete knowledge of the advantages, disadvantages, and individual needs of each patient before making a decision. This chapter will focus on graft options for ACL reconstruction, evaluating the existing literature in order to provide an up-to-date review on the subject and, hopefully, contribute to an evidence-based decision for graft choice in ACL reconstruction.

Keywords: ACL reconstruction, graft options, autograft, allograft, hamstring graft, quadriceps graft, patellar tendon graft

1. Introduction

Rupture of the anterior cruciate ligament (ACL) is a very common injury, especially in sports-related activities, with an annual incidence of 68.6 per 100,000 person-years [1]. Also, the number of surgeries being performed annually for an ACL tear has increased over the years. In the United States alone, the rates of ACL reconstruction have increased significantly in a 12-year period from 10.36 to 18.06 and from 22.58 to 25.42 per 100,000 person-years for females and males, respectively [2–4].

The gold standard treatment for active patients with ACL rupture consists in surgically reconstructing this ligament. The principle of this surgical intervention is to re-establish stability and function in the knee, preventing further damage of the knee joint [5].

Given the rise in ACL injuries and ACL reconstruction revision rates, there has been an increased interest in research, goal being to improve outcomes, decrease morbidity, and lower revision rates [2]. Various grafts are available for ACL reconstruction, including autografts [bone-patellar tendon-bone (BTB), hamstring tendon (HT), quadriceps tendon (QT)], allografts and synthetic grafts.

IntechOpen

The ideal graft for reconstruction of ACL is one which is biomechanically similar to the native ligament, can be easily harvested, has low harvest site morbidity, can be secured predictably, and gets well incorporated in the bone tunnels [3, 6]. When considering a graft source for the ACL reconstruction, the primary factor influencing a patient's decision is physician recommendation, hence the importance of a complete understanding of the graft options available [2, 7, 8].

2. Anatomy and function of the anterior cruciate ligament

The main function of the ACL is to provide anteroposterior and rotary stability to the knee. The ACL is the primary restraint to anterior translation of the tibia relative to the femur and is a major secondary restraint to internal rotation, particularly when the joint is near full extension [9].

It is composed of two functional bundles, based on their tibial insertion sites: the anteromedial (AM) and the posterolateral (PL) bundle [10]. These bundles function synergistically and have a distinct tensioning pattern throughout knee range of motion. When the knee is extended the PL bundle is tight, and the AM bundle is moderately lax. As the knee is flexed, the AM bundle tightens and the PL bundle loosens [11]. Also, biomechanical studies have shown that the PL bundle contributes the most to rotatory stability to the knee in lower degrees of flexion, and the anteromedial bundle provides more sagittal stability in higher degrees of flexion [2, 10]. In terms of dimensions, the ACL varies in length, ranging between 27 and 38 mm [12, 13]. There is also variability among individuals, in the femoral and tibial footprints of the ACL, with cross-sectional areas of 60–130 and 100–160 mm^2, respectively [12, 14, 15]. On average, the mid-substance of the ACL is 10 to 11 mm wide (range 7–17 mm) with an average thickness of 3.9 mm and a cross-sectional area of 40.9 ± 3 mm [2, 16].

Awareness of the overall dimensions of the native ACL, both the insertion sites and at its isthmus, is important when determining the size of the ACL graft and fixation angle during reconstruction [14].

With regard to structure, the ACL has a microstructure of collagen bundles of multiple types (mostly type I) and a matrix made of a network of proteins, glycoproteins, elastic systems, and glycosaminoglycans with multiple functional interactions [9]. Its sporadic fiber arrangement allows for a higher tensile strength than many other ligaments, with a maximum tensile strength reported as high as 2160 N (mean tensile strength approximately 1725 N), with a stiffness of 242 N/mm (mean stiffness 182 N/mm) and a strain rate of approximately 20% before failure [2, 17]. However, ultimate tensile load and linear stiffness decrease significantly with age: to 658 (129) N and 180 (25) N/mm, respectively, for older specimens (60–97 years) [9, 18].

3. Graft options

There are several options to consider when choosing a graft for ACL reconstruction. These options can be broken down to autografts, allografts, or synthetic grafts. The choice of graft should also be individualized to the patient's needs, anatomy, sport type, level of competition, and age. Another issue to consider is graft size, as it increases so does strength, but it also can lead to impingement with the notch and create arthrofibrosis [2, 19]. Recent studies have shown that graft size and tunnel positions should follow the patient's native anatomy in an attempt to reproduce and mimic the native ACL and improve long-term outcomes [20, 21]. It has been shown that anatomic ACL reconstructions reduce the risk of posttraumatic osteoarthritis (OA) at long-term follow-up [2, 22].

3.1 Autografts

Autografts are more commonly used than allografts and synthetic grafts [3]. In general, autografts are reported to have faster incorporation times, less failure rates overall, and no risk of disease transmission, but there is some morbidity with the graft harvest. Three main autografts are usually used: BTB, HT, and QT [2, 3, 23]. Furthermore, autografts are usually harvested from the ipsilateral extremity but can also be harvested from the uninjured knee. There are authors who advocate advantages of harvesting an autograft from the contralateral side [24].

3.1.1 Bone-patellar tendon-bone

BTB autograft (**Figure 1**) has historically served as the gold standard for ACL reconstruction mostly because of its long-standing track record and widespread use [2, 25]. The central third of the patellar tendon was also the first autograft option consistently used for ACL reconstruction [25]. One of the main advantages with this graft is that it allows fast bone to bone healing within the tibial and femoral tunnels [3]. Also, the clinical results reported are very good in terms of stability and return to play. The long-term results (17–20 years) have shown 83% of patients having stable, normal, or near-normal functions, and 1.6% of patients needed revision ACL reconstruction [3, 6]. More recent studies and meta-analyses have shown that BTB autografts have lower failure rates and higher return-to-sport rates compared with HT autografts, especially in the young athletic patient population [2, 26]. Some studies

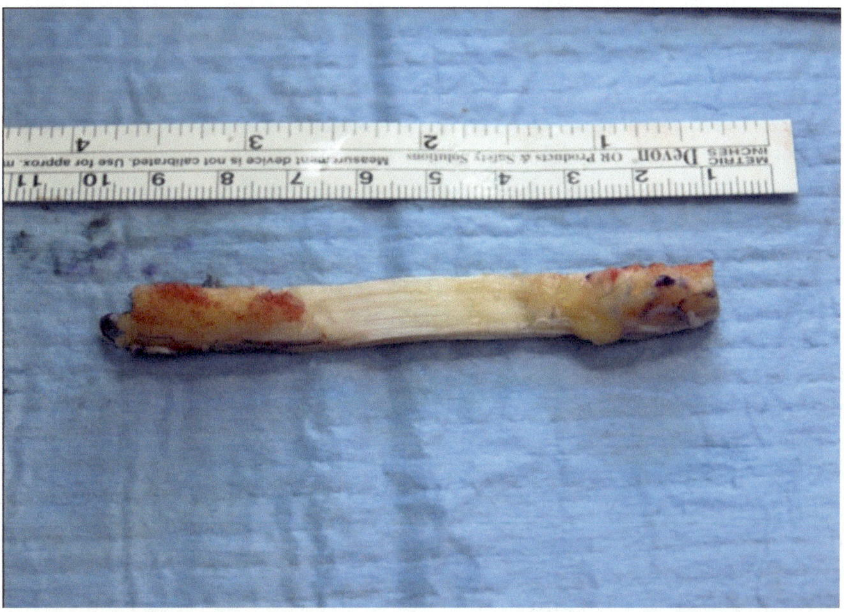

Figure 1.
BTB autograft.

have also found less residual anterior knee laxity and improved stability with the use of BTB autograft versus HT autograft at longer-term follow-up [26, 27].

Other long-term level I and II evidence studies comparing HT and BTB autografts have consistently shown no statistically significant difference in knee laxity [7, 28].

In terms of strength and stiffness, a 10-mm BTB graft has been found to resist to tensile loads of up to 2977 N with a stiffness of about 620 N/mm, numbers that exceed the strength and stiffness of the native ACL [29]. Donor site morbidity is another important aspect to consider when choosing a graft for ACL reconstruction.

In general, the patellar tendon graft is recognized as the graft with the highest harvest site morbidity, including anterior knee pain, kneeling pain, and patellar fracture [30]. If patellar fractures and patellar tendon ruptures are uncommon complications after BTB harvest, anterior knee pain has been frequently associated with BTB autograft use [2, 27, 30]. Some authors recommend that BTB graft for ACL reconstruction should be avoided in patients whose occupation or lifestyle requires frequent kneeling [3]. There is some evidence that anterior knee pain after ACL surgery may be more related to loss of motion and poor rehabilitation rather than graft choice, and studies have demonstrated a decrease in anterior knee symptoms after initiation of an accelerated rehabilitation program that emphasizes knee extension [2, 17]. Mismatch of BTB graft and tunnel length may also lead to a small tibial bone plug and compromise the strength of the fixation [31]. BTB autograft is also contraindicated in skeletally immature individuals as the graft harvest and fixation methods would violate the physes and increase the risk of growth arrest [2]. On the other hand, revision surgery, after a failed ACL reconstruction with BTB graft, may be easier as tunnel enlargement is not usually encountered as bone-to-bone healing prevents tunnel widening.

3.1.2 Hamstring tendons

HT autografts are currently the most popular graft choice for ACL reconstruction, having some key advantages. The semitendinosus tendon is the main graft that can be harvested with or without the gracilis tendon, usually from the ipsilateral leg. One attractive point is the minimally invasive nature of the harvest, thus minimizing donor site morbidity [3, 6]. Hamstring grafts are associated with lower risk of long-term anterior knee pain compared to BTB grafts [31]. Other advantages have been reported with the use of HT, including greater cross-sectional area, avoidance of the extensor mechanism in the graft harvesting process, and that it is an option for ACL reconstruction in the skeletally immature [2, 32].

With regard to strength and stiffness, a 4-strand HT graft has a tensile load of up to 4000 N with a stiffness of about 750 N/mm [33].

Clinical results are also good, but some studies are indicating more failures compared to BTB. In a meta-analysis in 2007, Poolman et al. showed reduced morbidity using HT autograft for ACL reconstruction. Authors stated that the modern endobutton hamstring graft fixation technique (two studies) yielded similar stability in the Lachman test as BTB grafts [34]. Another meta-analysis by Biau et al. from 6 published randomized clinical trials which included 423 patients with symptomatic unilateral ACL injury randomly assigned to reconstruction with patellar tendon or HT autograft showed postoperative knee instability was less common after ACL reconstruction with patellar tendon autograft than with HT autograft [35]. The difference was noted especially with the pivot-shift and for females and younger patients. Reinhardt et al. showed in systematic review, a graft failure rate lower for BTB than for HT (7.2 vs.

15.8%, respectively) (p = .02) [36]. Magnussen et al. showed, in a systematic review, graft failure lower for BTB compared to HT but without statistical significance [37]. There was no difference in patient-reported outcomes (IKDC). Anterior knee pain and kneeling pain were higher for BTB. More recently, in 2015, Xie et al. showed no difference in re-tear rate between patellar tendon and hamstrings and no difference for patient-reported outcome measures. However, reconstruction with patellar tendon graft resulted in better rotational stability and return to preinjury level of activity. Again, anterior knee pain and kneeling pain were greater for BTB [38].

Disadvantages associated with HT grafts include prolonged healing times, unpredictable graft size, higher failure rates in certain patient populations, and knee flexion weakness [2, 32]. The latter, risk of residual hamstring weakness, makes the graft a relative contraindication for athletes who need power in flexion for their athletic performance (i.e., sprinters, judo wrestlers) [2]. However, the main concern after HT autograft ACL reconstruction is graft failure. In particular, HT autograft seems to fail more among younger female patients, with graft rupture reported at 17.5% after HT autograft compared with 6.4% after BTB autograft in females aged 15 to 20 years [2, 39].

HT grafts less than 8 mm in diameter are a risk factor for poor patient outcomes, with an increase in failure rates, particularly in patients younger than 20 years [40]. This is of particular importance in hamstring autograft procedures because hamstring tendons, specifically in younger female population, tend to be insufficient and more prone to failure [41, 42]. Therefore, to address this issue, techniques that involve increasing hamstring graft thickness by folding the graft on top of itself have been developed [42]. The usual preparation technique for a HT graft is a doubled semitendinosus and gracilis resulting in a four-strand configuration as shown in **Figure 2** [43]. Another popular technique, in order to obtain a thicker graft, is a five-strand configuration, with a tripled semitendinosus and a doubled gracilis [42]. There is also the option of using a single tendon, usually the semitendinosus, in a 3- or 4-strand configuration. This technique can also be used with two suspensory devices for an all-inside ACL reconstruction [42, 44].

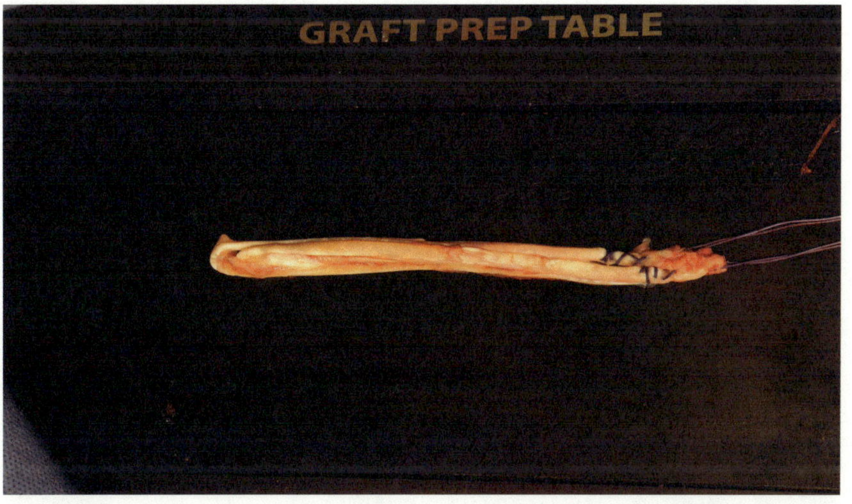

Figure 2.
Four-strand HT graft.

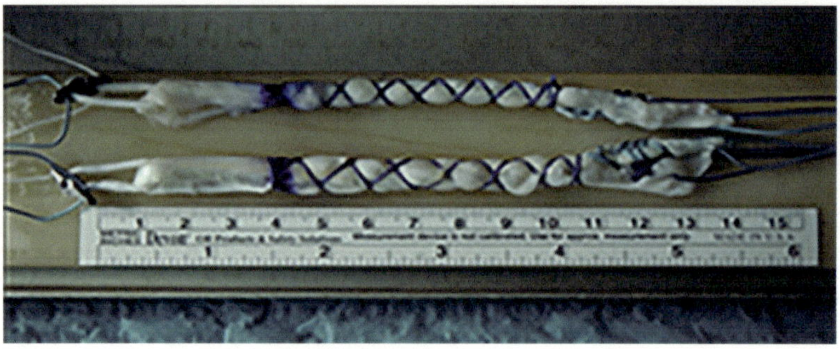

Figure 3.
HT graft prepared for a double-bundle ACL reconstruction.

HT grafts can be prepared as two individual grafts making the construct suitable for a double-bundle ACL reconstruction; the PL bundle is reconstructed using a double gracilis, and the AM bundle is reconstructed with a doubled semitendinosus (**Figure 3**).

3.1.3 Quadriceps tendon

The QT graft (**Figure 4**) is the least popular autograft source but has gained much attention in the last few years [45]. There are some important advantages reported with this graft, making it more and more appealing for ACL reconstruction. Among the proposed advantages are low morbidity at the harvest site [46, 47], predictable size and great versatility, the ability to harvest grafts in different widths, thicknesses, and lengths [23]. It can be harvested with or without a bone block as well as a full or partial thickness graft [48]. QT is a reliable and robust graft with a cross-sectional area up to twice that of a BTB autograft [2, 49]. The graft is longer and wider, has a higher tensile strength, about 50% more mass than a BTB autograft, and has been shown to be biomechanically similar to the six-strand HT autograft with regard to ultimate load to failure [2, 50]. It is also suitable for double-bundle ACL reconstruction [51]. The free quadriceps graft eliminates the risk of patella fracture and is also suitable for pediatric patients [52] (video link here).

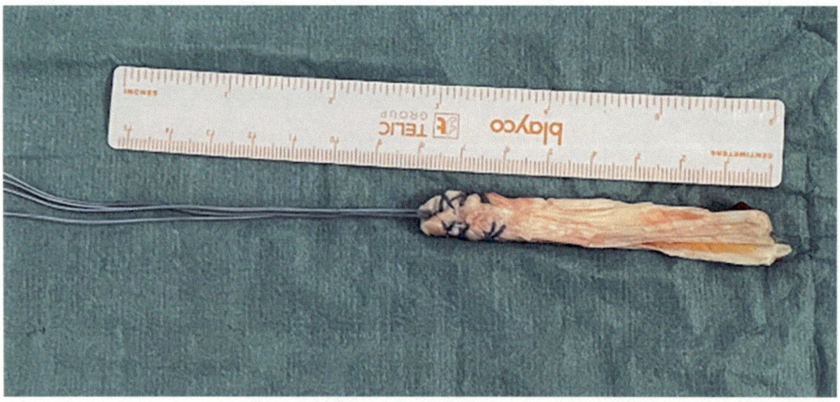

Figure 4.
QT graft – Without a bone block.

The available data on QT for ACL reconstruction are limited, at least compared to HT and BTB grafts. Nonetheless, clinical results are promising. Lund et al. found no difference in anterior knee pain and functional outcomes in a prospective randomized trial comparing QT with patellar tendon. However, knee walking pain was significantly less for QT than with BTB [53]. A systematic review by Slone et al. in 2014 showed no difference for stability, range of motion, functional outcomes, and complications between quadriceps graft and BTB. Also, less donor site morbidity was found for QT [45]. A retrospective study by Geib et al. compared QT autografts with 30 BTB autograft reconstructions. The QT graft group was found to have a significantly lower percentage of knees with greater than 3 mm of side-to-side laxity on arthrometer testing when compared with the BTB group; however, no significant differences were found between the two groups on Lachman and pivot-shift testing [54]. A more recent meta-analysis evaluating 27 clinical studies with 2856 patients (Level of Evidence II) concluded that QT had similar graft survival rates and comparable functional and clinical outcomes when compared with BTB and HT autografts [2, 55]. QT also showed improved functional outcomes compared with HT autograft and significantly less harvest site pain compared with BTB autograft. A registry-based study did show a higher revision rate for QT (4.7%) versus HT and BTB (2.3% versus 1.5%, respectively), although QT patients in this study comprised only 3.2% of the patient sample and graft size, fixation technique, and bone block use were not available for analysis [2, 56].

3.2 Allograft

The main reason for allograft choice is the complete avoidance of graft harvest morbidity. Other advantages of allografts over autografts are shorter surgical times, predictable graft size, and easier recovery in the immediate postoperative period [2, 6]. Disadvantages include disease transmission, immunogenic response, weakening of graft tissues that occurs due to sterilization and processing techniques, and slower incorporation times [2, 3, 57, 58]. Also, the increased cost is another downside of using allografts, and they are not as widely available in other countries outside of the United States [2, 6].

The commonly used allografts for ACL reconstruction are BTB grafts, HT grafts, tibialis posterior/anterior, peroneal tendons, iliotibial band, and Achilles tendon [2, 6].

Allografts are prepared using deep freezing, radiation, chlorhexidine, or supercritical carbon dioxide, with these processing techniques affecting the overall structural and mechanical properties of allografts to varying extents, with inferior outcomes reported in irradiated and chemically processed allografts [31, 59]. Irradiated allografts are more likely to fail because of decreased mechanical properties due to sterilization and possibility of triggering an inflammatory response [3, 6]. The use of fresh frozen and non-irradiated allografts is reported to improve graft survival rates and could be a better option compared to irradiated allografts [31].

Regarding outcomes after ACL reconstruction with allograft, studies have consistently shown that allografts have a higher re-rupture rate than autografts in young, athletic individuals [2, 60]. Wasserstein et al. showed that in active patients aged <25 years, there was a 9.6% graft rupture rate with autograft versus 25.0% with allograft [61]. Another study found the use of allografts in primary ACL reconstruction to be associated with a 5.2 times greater risk of graft rupture compared to BTB autografts ($P < 0.01$), and patients under 30 years of age to be associated with increased risk of re-rupture [31, 60]. The study reported that by mid-30 years of age, there was no difference in graft rupture rate by graft choice. Even more studies have demonstrated that outcomes and revision rates after allograft use in patients who are aged >40 years are consistently similar to those after autograft ACL reconstructions [2, 62]. Recently, allograft use in young active patients is recognized as a risk factor for retear; graft choice by surgeons changed in the late period to use of allografts in older and less-active patients, which correlated with a significant decrease in retear risk [63]. Also, studies have shown slower incorporation times, revascularization, and "ligamentization" of allografts compared to autografts [64, 65]. However, this aspect alone does not explain the higher failure rates of allografts compared to autografts seen mainly in the young athletic population and not in the older, less demanding patients. Looking at the available data, the answer could be found in the sterilization process and the rehabilitation program. For example, in the study by Wasserstein et al. [61] who reported, on seven studies addressing patients aged less than 25 years, higher failure rates of allografts versus autografts, only two studies assessed autograft versus non-irradiated allograft, and in this analysis no statistically significant difference in graft failure was seen. Liu et al. [66] showed, in a recent systematic review, that non-irradiated allografts are superior to irradiated allografts based on improved knee joint functional scores and decreased failure rate. Also, Wang et al. [67] performed a meta-analysis looking at autograft versus non-irradiated and irradiated allografts. A total of 1172 patients were involved with mean patient age varying from 22 to 32.8 years. Although autograft offered greater advantages in functional outcomes and adverse events than irradiated allograft in ACL reconstruction, there were no significant differences between autograft and non-irradiated allograft in ACL reconstruction. On the other hand, other studies still show a higher failure rate in young patients treated with allograft tissue even with non-irradiated allografts [68]. Another theory that could explain higher rates of failure of allografts in younger patients is looking at rehabilitation. Mainly, donor site morbidity from graft harvest is eliminated when using allograft and patients are tempted to push the boundaries of their rehabilitation [69].

Another important role for allografts is revision ACL surgery. Large allografts, such as Achilles or QT, afford the additional advantage of a large cross-sectional area to fill large tunnels, have favorable time-zero biomechanical strength, and have a bone plug for bone-to-bone healing and fixation in at least a single tunnel. A study of the epidemiology of the Multicenter ACL Revision Study (MARS) cohort demonstrated that 54% of the surgeons used an allograft at the time of revision compared with 27% of the patients having had an allograft at the time of their primary reconstruction [70]. Also, multi-ligament knee surgery is another common scenario for the use of allograft tissue. Allograft use is appealing in multi-ligament knee injuries because of the need for multiple grafts to be available, the poor condition of the autograft tissues, and the attempt to limit further damage to the patient by harvesting autografts [71].

3.3 Synthetic grafts

Synthetic grafts have been developed in an attempt to overcome the concerns and disadvantages with auto- and allografts. They became popular in 1980 and early 1990, but the initial enthusiasm was soon discarded as early generations synthetic grafts failed.

The Ligament Augment Reconstruction System (LARS) (Surgical Implants and Devices, Arc-sur-Tille, France) is a synthetic ligament scaffold composed of polyethylene terephthalate fibers. Chen et al. conducted a prospective cohort study in patients undergoing ACL reconstruction with HT autografts (n = 73) versus LARS (n = 38) with 10 years follow-up [31, 72]. The study showed no significant difference in ACL reconstruction with HT autograft and LARS group with respect to the graft failure, mean SSD difference, and overall IKDC score. Early subjective evaluation at 6 months showed improved outcomes in the LARS group compared to the HT autograft group. The authors concluded that primary ACL reconstruction using either synthetics with remnant preservation or hamstring autografts showed satisfactory outcomes, especially the long-term cumulative failure rate, at 10 years postoperatively. Patient-reported outcomes suggested that symptom relief and restoration of function might occur earlier in those with synthetics [72].

Also, the systematic review by Batty et al. presented data on the functional outcomes, complications, and patient-reported outcomes of synthetic grafts in cruciate ligament reconstruction [73]. The results of this systematic review suggest that the current synthetic designs do achieve a number of their intended goals, allowing restoration of knee stability and potentially a faster progression through postoperative rehabilitation. In the LARS ACL group, return to unrestricted sports was allowed between 2 and 6 months postoperatively. The authors also concluded that objective knee instability occurs at a rate of between 6% and 12% for the LARS. Earlier synthetic ligament device designs have higher rates of failure and rates of synovitis/sterile effusion. Results for newer-generation devices, specifically the LARS, appear to show lower reported rates of failure, revision, and sterile effusion/synovitis when compared with older devices. A limitation of this review is the paucity of well-conducted clinical trials included. In relation to the LARS device, there was only one RCT, so the results should therefore be interpreted with caution.

Currently used synthetic grafts for ACL reconstruction are ligament augmentation system (LARS and Leeds-Keio), augmentation being the key word. However, their use remains controversial [31].

4. Conclusion

There are many choices when it comes to graft selection for ACL reconstruction, and numerous patients and surgical factors contribute to selection of an ideal graft. The decision should be individualized to best match the patient's anatomy, age, needs, and expectations. It is important for surgeons to understand the best available evidence on graft choice. Based on the current literature, autograft seems to be superior to allograft with respect to graft failure, patient-reported outcomes, and return to sport in young, active patients. The most commonly used autografts for ACL reconstruction provide similar functional outcomes. BTB grafts are associated with more anterior knee pain and kneeling pain but have faster incorporation times and are still being accepted as the "gold standard" by some authors.

HT offers certain theoretical advantages in the subgroup of patients that do a lot of kneeling, with preexisting patellofemoral pain, patella alta, or in those with open physes. On the other hand, HT grafts may have slightly higher failure rates, especially when less than 8 mm in diameter; however, this could theoretically be managed by technical aspects like the 5–6 strands grafts. Also, potential hamstring weakness might be a concern in athletes.

QT seems to be a very versatile graft. In general, the results are similar with BTB but with less donor site morbidity.

Allografts should be used with caution in young athletes as they are reported to be a risk factor for graft failure in this group of patients. However, this risk appears to be mitigated to some extent with the use of fresh frozen non-irradiated allografts, with frequent use in the United States. Also, allograft plays an important role in patients over 35–40 years, in revision ACL reconstruction, and in multi-ligament knee injuries.

Synthetic grafts are still under evolution, and no perfect synthetic graft is available till date. However, a clear indication for the use of synthetic graft is ligament augmentation or bracing.

The treating surgeon should thus be familiar with all the ACL reconstruction options available to individualize and optimize each patient's treatment and outcomes.

Author details

Adrian Todor
Iuliu Hatieganu University of Medicine and Pharmacy, Department of Orthopedics, Traumatology and Pediatric Orthopedics, Cluj Napoca, Romania

*Address all correspondence to: adi.todor@yahoo.com

References

[1] Sanders TL, Maradit Kremers H, Bryan AJ, Larson DR, Dahm DL, Levy BA, et al. Incidence of anterior cruciate ligament tears and reconstruction: A 21-year population-based study. The American Journal of Sports Medicine. 2016;**44**(6):1502-1507. DOI: 10.1177/0363546516629944

[2] Buerba RA, Boden SA, Lesniak B. Graft selection in contemporary anterior cruciate ligament reconstruction. JAAOS Global Research & Reviews. 2021;**5**(10):e21.00230. DOI: 10.5435/JAAOSGlobal-D-21-00230

[3] Dhammi IK, Rehan-Ul-Haq, Kumar S. Graft choices for anterior cruciate ligament reconstruction. Indian Journal of Orthopaedics. 2015;**49**(2):127-128. DOI: 10.4103/0019-5413.152393

[4] Mall NA, Chalmers PN, Moric M, Tanaka MJ, Cole BJ, Bach BR Jr, et al. Incidence and trends of anterior cruciate ligament reconstruction in the United States. The American Journal of Sports Medicine. 2014;**42**(10):2363-2370. DOI: 10.1177/0363546514542796

[5] Fleaca R, Prejbeanu R, Feier AM, Russu O, Todor A, Predescu V, et al. Single- or double-bundle technique in the anterior cruciate ligament reconstruction – Current concepts and review of the literature. Journal of Interdisciplinary Medicine. 2016;**1**(S2):8-12. DOI: 10.1515/jim-2016-0047

[6] Chechik O, Amar E, Khashan M, Lador R, Eyal G, Gold A. An international survey on anterior cruciate ligament reconstruction practices. International Orthopaedics. 2013;**37**(2):201-206. DOI: 10.1007/s00264-012-1611-9

[7] Macaulay AA, Perfetti DC, Levine WN. Anterior cruciate ligament graft choices. Sports Health. 2012;**4**(1):63-68. DOI: 10.1177/1941738111409890

[8] Cohen SB, Yucha DT, Ciccotti MC, Goldstein DT, Ciccotti MA, Ciccotti MG. Factors affecting patient selection of graft type in anterior cruciate ligament reconstruction. Arthroscopy. 2009;**25**(9):1006-1010. DOI: 10.1016/j.arthro.2009.02.010

[9] Kraeutler MJ, Wolsky RM, Vidal AF, Bravman JT. Anatomy and biomechanics of the native and reconstructed anterior cruciate ligament: Surgical implications. The Journal of Bone and Joint Surgery. American Volume. 2017;**99**(5):438-445. DOI: 10.2106/JBJS.16.00754

[10] Duthon VB, Barea C, Abrassart S, Fasel JH, Fritschy D, Ménétrey J. Anatomy of the anterior cruciate ligament. Knee Surgery, Sports Traumatology, Arthroscopy. 2006;**14**(3):204-213. DOI: 10.1007/s00167-005-0679-9

[11] Zantop T, Herbort M, Raschke MJ, Fu FH, Petersen W. The role of the anteromedial and posterolateral bundles of the anterior cruciate ligament in anterior tibial translation and internal rotation. The American Journal of Sports Medicine. 2007;**35**(2):223-227. DOI: 10.1177/0363546506294571

[12] Fox MA, Engler ID, Zsidai BT, Hughes JD, Musahl V. Anatomic anterior cruciate ligament reconstruction: Freddie Fu's paradigm. Journal of ISAKOS. 2022;**S2059-7754**(22):00078-00075. DOI: 10.1016/j.jisako.2022.08.003

[13] Cone SG, Howe D, Fisher MB. Size and shape of the human anterior cruciate

ligament and the impact of sex and skeletal growth: A systematic review. JBJS Reviews. 2019;**7**(6):e8. DOI: 10.2106/JBJS.RVW.18.00145

[14] Iriuchishima T, Ryu K, Aizawa S, Fu FH. Size correlation between the tibial anterior cruciate ligament footprint and the tibia plateau. Knee Surgery, Sports Traumatology, Arthroscopy. 2015;**23**(4):1147-1152. DOI: 10.1007/s00167-014-2927-3

[15] Caterev S, Todor A, Khallouki Y, Bota NC, Zejly M, Nistor DV. Correlations between the anterior cruciate ligament insertion sites dimensions and patient's physical characteristics: An arthroscopic study. Chirurgia. 2018;**31**:5-9. DOI: 10.23736/S0394-9508.17.04739-8

[16] Cheung SC, Allen CR, Gallo RA, Ma CB, Feeley BT. Patients' attitudes and factors in their selection of grafts for anterior cruciate ligament reconstruction. The Knee. 2012;**19**(1):49-54. DOI: 10.1016/j.knee.2010.11.009

[17] West RV, Harner CD. Graft selection in anterior cruciate ligament reconstruction. The Journal of the American Academy of Orthopaedic Surgeons. 2005;**13**(3):197-207. DOI: 10.5435/00124635-200505000-00006

[18] Woo SL, Hollis JM, Adams DJ, Lyon RM, Takai S. Tensile properties of the human femur-anterior cruciate ligament-tibia complex. The effects of specimen age and orientation. The American Journal of Sports Medicine. 1991;**19**(3):217-225. DOI: 10.1177/036354659101900303

[19] Su AW, Storey EP, Lin SC, Forst B, Lawrence JT, Ganley TJ, et al. Association of the graft size and arthrofibrosis in young patients after primary anterior cruciate ligament reconstruction. The Journal of the American Academy of Orthopaedic Surgeons. 2018;**26**(23):e483-e489. DOI: 10.5435/JAAOS-D-17-00177

[20] Fu FH, van Eck CF, Tashman S, Irrgang JJ, Moreland MS. Anatomic anterior cruciate ligament reconstruction: A changing paradigm. Knee Surgery, Sports Traumatology, Arthroscopy. 2015;**23**(3):640-648. DOI: 10.1007/s00167-014-3209-9

[21] van Eck CF, Lesniak BP, Schreiber VM, Fu FH. Anatomic single- and double-bundle anterior cruciate ligament reconstruction flowchart. Arthroscopy. 2010;**26**(2):258-268. DOI: 10.1016/j.arthro.2009.07.027

[22] Rothrauff BB, Jorge A, de Sa D, Kay J, Fu FH, Musahl V. Anatomic ACL reconstruction reduces risk of post-traumatic osteoarthritis: A systematic review with minimum 10-year follow-up. Knee Surgery, Sports Traumatology, Arthroscopy. 2020;**28**(4):1072-1084. DOI: 10.1007/s00167-019-05665-2

[23] Todor A, Caterev S, Nistor DV, Khallouki Y. Free bone plug quadriceps tendon harvest and suspensory button attachment for anterior cruciate ligament reconstruction. Arthroscopy Techniques. 2016;**5**(3):e541-e544. DOI: 10.1016/j.eats.2016.02.001

[24] Shelbourne KD, Beck MB, Gray T. Anterior cruciate ligament reconstruction with contralateral autogenous patellar tendon graft: Evaluation of donor site strength and subjective results. The American Journal of Sports Medicine. 2015;**43**(3):648-653. DOI: 10.1177/0363546514560877

[25] Duchman KR, Lynch TS, Spindler KP. Graft selection in anterior cruciate ligament surgery: Who gets what

and why? Clinics in Sports Medicine. 2017;**36**(1):25-33. DOI: 10.1016/j.csm.2016.08.013

[26] Samuelsen BT, Webster KE, Johnson NR, Hewett TE, Krych AJ. Hamstring autograft versus patellar tendon autograft for ACL reconstruction: Is there a difference in graft failure rate? A meta-analysis of 47,613 patients. Clinical Orthopaedics and Related Research. 2017;**475**(10):2459-2468. DOI: 10.1007/s11999-017-5278-9

[27] Freedman KB, D'Amato MJ, Nedeff DD, Kaz A, Bach BR Jr. Arthroscopic anterior cruciate ligament reconstruction: A metaanalysis comparing patellar tendon and hamstring tendon autografts. The American Journal of Sports Medicine. 2003;**31**(1):2-11. DOI: 10.1177/03635465030310011501

[28] Holm I, Oiestad BE, Risberg MA, Aune AK. No difference in knee function or prevalence of osteoarthritis after reconstruction of the anterior cruciate ligament with 4-strand hamstring autograft versus patellar tendon-bone autograft: A randomized study with 10-year follow-up. The American Journal of Sports Medicine. 2010;**38**(3):448-454. DOI: 10.1177/0363546509350301

[29] Cooper DE, Deng XH, Burstein AL, Warren RF. The strength of the central third patellar tendon graft. A biomechanical study. The American Journal of Sports Medicine. 1993;**21**(6):818-823; discussion 823-4. DOI: 10.1177/036354659302100610

[30] Milankov M, Kecojević V, Rasović P, Kovacević N, Gvozdenović N, Obradović M. Disruption of the knee extensor apparatus complicating anterior cruciate ligament reconstruction. Acta Chirurgica Iugoslavica. 2013;**60**(2):13-21. DOI: 10.2298/aci1302013m

[31] Baawa-Ameyaw J, Plastow R, Begum FA, Kayani B, Jeddy H, Haddad F. Current concepts in graft selection for anterior cruciate ligament reconstruction. EFORT Open Reviews. 2021;**6**(9):808-815. DOI: 10.1302/2058-5241.6.210023

[32] Cerulli G, Placella G, Sebastiani E, Tei MM, Speziali A, Manfreda F. ACL reconstruction: Choosing the graft. Joints. 2013;**1**(1):18-24

[33] Hamner DL, Brown CH Jr, Steiner ME, Hecker AT, Hayes WC. Hamstring tendon grafts for reconstruction of the anterior cruciate ligament: Biomechanical evaluation of the use of multiple strands and tensioning techniques. The Journal of Bone and Joint Surgery. American Volume. 1999;**81**(4):549-557. DOI: 10.2106/00004623-199904000-00013

[34] Poolman RW, Farrokhyar F, Bhandari M. Hamstring tendon autograft better than bone patellar-tendon bone autograft in ACL reconstruction: A cumulative meta-analysis and clinically relevant sensitivity analysis applied to a previously published analysis. Acta Orthopaedica. 2007;**78**(3):350-354. DOI: 10.1080/17453670710013915

[35] Biau DJ, Katsahian S, Kartus J, Harilainen A, Feller JA, Sajovic M, et al. Patellar tendon versus hamstring tendon autografts for reconstructing the anterior cruciate ligament: A meta-analysis based on individual patient data. The American Journal of Sports Medicine. 2009;**37**(12):2470-2478. DOI: 10.1177/0363546509333006

[36] Reinhardt KR, Hetsroni I, Marx RG. Graft selection for anterior cruciate ligament reconstruction: A level I systematic review comparing failure rates and functional outcomes. The

Orthopedic Clinics of North America. 2010;**41**(2):249-262. DOI: 10.1016/j.ocl.2009.12.009

[37] Magnussen RA, Carey JL, Spindler KP. Does autograft choice determine intermediate-term outcome of ACL reconstruction? Knee Surgery, Sports Traumatology, Arthroscopy. 2011;**19**(3):462-472. DOI: 10.1007/s00167-010-1277-z

[38] Xie X, Liu X, Chen Z, Yu Y, Peng S, Li Q. A meta-analysis of bone-patellar tendon-bone autograft versus four-strand hamstring tendon autograft for anterior cruciate ligament reconstruction. The Knee. 2015;**22**(2):100-110. DOI: 10.1016/j.knee.2014.11.014

[39] Salem HS, Varzhapetyan V, Patel N, Dodson CC, Tjoumakaris FP, Freedman KB. Anterior cruciate ligament reconstruction in young female athletes: Patellar versus hamstring tendon autografts. The American Journal of Sports Medicine. 2019;**47**(9):2086-2092. DOI: 10.1177/0363546519854762

[40] Iriuchishima T, Shirakura K, Yorifuji H, Aizawa S, Fu FH. Size comparison of ACL footprint and reconstructed auto graft. Knee Surgery, Sports Traumatology, Arthroscopy. 2013;**21**(4):797-803. DOI: 10.1007/s00167-012-1949-y

[41] Barrett GR, Noojin FK, Hartzog CW, Nash CR. Reconstruction of the anterior cruciate ligament in females: A comparison of hamstring versus patellar tendon autograft. Arthroscopy. 2002;**18**(1):46-54. DOI: 10.1053/jars.2002.25974

[42] Vinagre G, Kennedy NI, Chahla J, Cinque ME, Hussain ZB, Olesen ML, et al. Hamstring graft preparation techniques for anterior cruciate ligament reconstruction. Arthroscopy Techniques. 2017;**6**(6):e2079-e2084. DOI: 10.1016/j.eats.2017.08.031

[43] Brown CH Jr. Editorial commentary: How to increase hamstring tendon graft size for anterior cruciate ligament reconstruction. Arthroscopy. 2018;**34**(9):2641-2646. DOI: 10.1016/j.arthro.2018.06.014

[44] Lubowitz JH. All-inside anterior cruciate ligament graft link: Graft preparation technique. Arthroscopy Techniques. 2012;**1**(2):e165-e168. DOI: 10.1016/j.eats.2012.06.002

[45] Diermeier T, Tisherman R, Hughes J, Tulman M, Baum Coffey E, Fink C, et al. Quadriceps tendon anterior cruciate ligament reconstruction. Knee Surgery, Sports Traumatology, Arthroscopy. 2020;**28**(8):2644-2656. DOI: 10.1007/s00167-020-05902-z

[46] Slone HS, Romine SE, Premkumar A, Xerogeanes JW. Quadriceps tendon autograft for anterior cruciate ligament reconstruction: A comprehensive review of current literature and systematic review of clinical results. Arthroscopy. 2015;**31**(3):541-554. DOI: 10.1016/j.arthro.2014.11.010

[47] Buescu CT, Onutu AH, Lucaciu DO, Todor A. Pain level after ACL reconstruction: A comparative study between free quadriceps tendon and hamstring tendons autografts. Acta Orthopaedica et Traumatologica Turcica. 2017;**51**(2):100-103. DOI: 10.1016/j.aott.2017.02.011

[48] Rabuck SJ, Musahl V, Fu FH, West RV. Anatomic anterior cruciate ligament reconstruction with quadriceps tendon autograft. Clinics in Sports Medicine. 2013;**32**(1):155-164. DOI: 10.1016/j.csm.2012.08.014

[49] Shani RH, Umpierez E, Nasert M, Hiza EA, Xerogeanes J. Biomechanical

comparison of quadriceps and patellar tendon grafts in anterior cruciate ligament reconstruction. Arthroscopy. 2016;**32**(1):71-75. DOI: 10.1016/j.arthro.2015.06.051

[50] Musahl V, Karlsson J. Anterior cruciate ligament tear. The New England Journal of Medicine. 2019;**380**(24):2341-2348. DOI: 10.1056/NEJMcp1805931

[51] Caterev S, Nistor DV, Todor A. Anatomic double-bundle anterior cruciate ligament reconstruction with a free quadriceps tendon autograft. Arthroscopy Techniques. 2016;**5**(5):e1063-e1067. DOI: 10.1016/j.eats.2016.05.015

[52] Marx RG, Hsu J, Fink C, Eriksson K, Vincent A, van der Merwe WM. Graft choices for pediatric anterior cruciate ligament reconstruction: State of the art. Journal of ISAKOS. 2023;**S2059-7754**(23):00001-00009. DOI: 10.1016/j.jisako.2023.01.001

[53] Lund B, Nielsen T, Faunø P, Christiansen SE, Lind M. Is quadriceps tendon a better graft choice than patellar tendon? A prospective randomized study. Arthroscopy. 2014;**30**(5):593-598. DOI: 10.1016/j.arthro.2014.01.012

[54] Geib TM, Shelton WR, Phelps RA, Clark L. Anterior cruciate ligament reconstruction using quadriceps tendon autograft: Intermediate-term outcome. Arthroscopy. 2009;**25**(12):1408-1414. DOI: 10.1016/j.arthro.2009.06.004

[55] Mouarbes D, Menetrey J, Marot V, Courtot L, Berard E, Cavaignac E. Anterior cruciate ligament reconstruction: A systematic review and meta-analysis of outcomes for quadriceps tendon autograft versus bone-patellar tendon-bone and hamstring-tendon autografts. The American Journal of Sports Medicine. 2019;**47**(14):3531-3540. DOI: 10.1177/0363546518825340

[56] Lind M, Strauss MJ, Nielsen T, Engebretsen L. Quadriceps tendon autograft for anterior cruciate ligament reconstruction is associated with high revision rates: Results from the Danish knee ligament registry. Knee Surgery, Sports Traumatology, Arthroscopy. 2020;**28**(7):2163-2169. DOI: 10.1007/s00167-019-05751-5

[57] Hu J, Qu J, Xu D, Zhou J, Lu H. Allograft versus autograft for anterior cruciate ligament reconstruction: An up-to-date meta-analysis of prospective studies. International Orthopaedics. 2013;**37**(2):311-320. DOI: 10.1007/s00264-012-1720-5

[58] Vyas D, Rabuck SJ, Harner CD. Allograft anterior cruciate ligament reconstruction: Indications, techniques, and outcomes. The Journal of Orthopaedic and Sports Physical Therapy. 2012;**42**(3):196-207. DOI: 10.2519/jospt.2012.4083

[59] Sun K, Tian S, Zhang J, Xia C, Zhang C, Yu T. Anterior cruciate ligament reconstruction with BPTB autograft, irradiated versus non-irradiated allograft: A prospective randomized clinical study. Knee Surgery, Sports Traumatology, Arthroscopy. 2009;**17**(5):464-474. DOI: 10.1007/s00167-008-0714-8

[60] Kaeding CC, Pedroza AD, Reinke EK, Huston LJ, Hewett TE, Flanigan DC, et al. Change in anterior cruciate ligament graft choice and outcomes over time. Arthroscopy. 2017;**33**(11):2007-2014. DOI: 10.1016/j.arthro.2017.06.019

[61] Wasserstein D, Sheth U, Cabrera A, Spindler KP. A systematic review of failed anterior cruciate ligament reconstruction with autograft compared with allograft in young patients. Sports Health. 2015;**7**(3):207-216. DOI: 10.1177/1941738115579030

[62] Maletis GB, Chen J, Inacio MC, Funahashi TT. Age-related risk factors for revision anterior cruciate ligament reconstruction: A cohort study of 21,304 patients from the Kaiser Permanente anterior cruciate ligament registry. The American Journal of Sports Medicine. 2016;**44**(2):331-336. DOI: 10.1177/0363546515614813

[63] Kaeding CC, Pedroza AD, Reinke EK, Huston LJ, MOON Consortium, Spindler KP. Risk factors and predictors of subsequent ACL injury in either knee after ACL reconstruction: Prospective analysis of 2488 primary ACL reconstructions from the MOON cohort. The American Journal of Sports Medicine. 2015;**43**(7):1583-1590. DOI: 10.1177/0363546515578836

[64] Scheffler SU, Schmidt T, Gangéy I, Dustmann M, Unterhauser F, Weiler A. Fresh-frozen free-tendon allografts versus autografts in anterior cruciate ligament reconstruction: Delayed remodeling and inferior mechanical function during long-term healing in sheep. Arthroscopy. 2008;**24**(4):448-458. DOI: 10.1016/j.arthro.2007.10.011

[65] Muramatsu K, Hachiya Y, Izawa H. Serial evaluation of human anterior cruciate ligament grafts by contrast-enhanced magnetic resonance imaging: Comparison of allografts and autografts. Arthroscopy. 2008;**24**(9):1038-1044. DOI: 10.1016/j.arthro.2008.05.014

[66] Liu Y, Liu X, Liu Y, Yang S. Comparison of clinical outcomes of using the nonirradiated and irradiated allograft for anterior cruciate ligament (ACL) reconstruction: A systematic review update and meta-analysis. Medicine (Baltimore). 2022;**101**(32):e29990. DOI: 10.1097/MD.0000000000029990

[67] Wang S, Zhang C, Cai Y, Lin X. Autograft or allograft? Irradiated or not? A contrast between autograft and allograft in anterior cruciate ligament reconstruction: A meta-analysis. Arthroscopy. 2018;**34**(12):3258-3265. DOI: 10.1016/j.arthro.2018.06.053

[68] Kane PW, Wascher J, Dodson CC, Hammoud S, Cohen SB, Ciccotti MG. Anterior cruciate ligament reconstruction with bone-patellar tendon-bone autograft versus allograft in skeletally mature patients aged 25 years or younger. Knee Surgery, Sports Traumatology, Arthroscopy. 2016;**24**(11):3627-3633. DOI: 10.1007/s00167-016-4213-z

[69] Hulet C, Sonnery-Cottet B, Stevenson C, Samuelsson K, Laver L, Zdanowicz U, et al. The use of allograft tendons in primary ACL reconstruction. Knee Surgery, Sports Traumatology, Arthroscopy. 2019;**27**(6):1754-1770. DOI: 10.1007/s00167-019-05440-3

[70] MARS Group, Wright RW, Huston LJ, Spindler KP, Dunn WR, Haas AK, et al. Descriptive epidemiology of the Multicenter ACL revision study (MARS) cohort. The American Journal of Sports Medicine. 2010;**38**(10):1979-1986. DOI: 10.1177/0363546510378645

[71] Strauss MJ, Varatojo R, Boutefnouchet T, Condello V, Samuelsson K, Gelber PE, et al. The use of allograft tissue in posterior cruciate, collateral and multi-ligament knee reconstruction. Knee Surgery, Sports Traumatology, Arthroscopy. 2019;**27**(6):1791-1809. DOI: 10.1007/s00167-019-05426-1

[72] Chen T, Zhang P, Chen J, Hua Y, Chen S. Long-term outcomes of anterior cruciate ligament reconstruction using either synthetics with remnant preservation or hamstring autografts: A 10-year longitudinal study. The American Journal of Sports

Medicine. 2017;**45**(12):2739-2750. DOI: 10.1177/0363546517721692

[73] Batty LM, Norsworthy CJ, Lash NJ, Wasiak J, Richmond AK, Feller JA. Synthetic devices for reconstructive surgery of the cruciate ligaments: A systematic review. Arthroscopy. 2015;**31**(5):957-968. DOI: 10.1016/j.arthro.2014.11.032

Chapter 5

Hidden Lesions of the Knee: Meniscal Ramp Lesions

Iffath Misbah, Girinivasan Chellamuthu and Munis Ashraf

Abstract

Meniscal RAMP lesions are not uncommon with ACL injuries and their incidence is higher in young males sustaining non-contact injuries. Diagnosis requires awareness of the lesion, and its hidden location and how to access it on arthroscopy remain the gold standard in detecting these tears. Despite trials to explain RAMP lesions by signal changes on MR imaging, a correlation was built in only one third of the cases. The healing potential along with the effect on knee stability of RAMP lesions is the reason behind repairing them. In this chapter, we intend to outline the description, incidence, effects, diagnosis and treatment outcomes of these lesions.

Keywords: RAMP, hidden lesions, MRI, treatment, rehabilitation

1. Introduction

The ramp in the posteromedial knee, the so-called because of its sheer resemblance to the ramps that we use to climb, is not a new structure to be described. However, there is a sudden surge in interest in addressing the lesions in this area—called the Ramp lesions. These lesions were described as early as 1983 by Hamberg et al. [1, 2]. Michael J. Strobel invented the term "Ramp lesion" to describe this disorder. He says that a meniscal injury known as a "ramp lesion," which obliterates the posterior horn of the medial meniscus's peripheral connection, commonly occurs in conjunction with an ACL tear [3].

Despite being a recognized entity for many years, these lesions were not considered important until recent years. The reasons are that these are the commonly missed lesions unless one is very particular—be it arthroscopically or in the MRIs. The knee is kept extended during the bulk of MRI processes. Ramp lesions are more difficult to analyse in this position because there is less space on the posterior and medial sides. One should be aware of the associated signs of ramp lesions like posteromedial tibial bone bruises. During the routine diagnostic arthroscopy of the knee, as emphasized by Sonnery-Cottet and his colleagues, 40 percent of these injuries are missed out. Only a trans-notch view may show these rips, allowing for a thorough assessment of the posteromedial compartment and a determination of the mobility of the posterior horn of the medial meniscus [4]. These characteristics have paved the way for these lesions to be called "hidden lesions" ultimately making them "forgotten lesions" for several years.

Since ACL reconstructions are among the most common knee operations, there has recently been a global search for surgical perfection. Due to recent research that

IntechOpen

suggests ramp lesions contribute to anterior and rotational stability, interest in them has been revived [5, 6].

The definition of Ramp lesions varies in the literature. But generally, they are described as longitudinal or oblique superior meniscocapsular junction tears or the tears in the meniscotibial ligament that typically occur in association with the ACL tears [4, 7]. These mediolateral tears are generally less than 2 cm [8].

2. Anatomy

The meniscotibial ligament attaches to the medial meniscus anteriorly, while the meniscocapsular expansion, also known as the meniscocapsular ligament, attaches to the medial meniscus posteriorly. Knowing the length of this area as well as how the meniscotibial ligaments and meniscocapsular junction adhere to the medial meniscus's back is absolutely crucial.

Based on its capsular attachment and degree of movement, the medial meniscus has been subdivided into a number of zones [9, 10]. The anterior root, also known as zone 1, the anteromedial zone, also known as zone 2, the medial zone, also known as zone 3, the Ramp area also known as zone 4 and the posterior zone, also known as zone 5, were the five zones identified by Smigielski et al. The band of fibrous connective tissue known as the meniscotibial ligament, commonly referred to as the coronary ligament, holds the meniscus to the tibia 7–10 mm below the articular surface, and the meniscotibial ligament is attached to the tibia. As a result of this association, a depression in the posterior femur develops at this location. These results contradict what was previously described for the ramp region by Diphillipo et al. [11]. The posterior zone of the medial meniscus contains descriptions of several attachments to the meniscocapsular and meniscotibial structures. The meniscocapsular ligament, also known as the meniscocapsular attachment, was 20.2 +/– 6 mm on average in length. This attachment was said to become conjoint with the meniscotibial ligament. Above the meniscocapsular ligament and below the superior border of the meniscus, this unified tissue joins to the posterior horn of the medial meniscus, creating a depression above the meniscus. This corresponds to the description of the posterior femoral recess by Smigielski et al. Implications for clinical practice arise from the fact that the ramp area may be reconnected to the posterior capsule after all-inside device repair of ramp lesions, thus bypassing the posterior femoral recess.

Because of its importance in ramp lesion pathophysiology, the architecture of the semimembranosus muscle, and more specifically its distal insertion, must be understood in order to grasp the mechanics of ramp lesions. The semimembranosus has its origin in the upper lateral facet of the ischial tuberosity. It has a complex insertion distally, described variedly across the literature. It is said to have 4 to 8 insertions. There are descriptions of three constant insertions. The lateral collateral ligament attaches inferiorly to the posteromedial tibia, anteriorly to the medial collateral ligament, and laterally to the oblique popliteal ligament and other anteromedial knee tissues, such as the medial meniscus [12]. The SANTI group also noticed the Semimembranosus Capsular Branch, which connects the semimembranosus muscle to the posterior capsule of the knee [13]. This capsular limb is important for understanding the mechanics of ramp fractures. In the literature, it has been reported that the semimembranosus tendon does not directly pass through the posterior horn of the medial meniscus. At best, there is a shaky connection between them. The meniscotibial ligament and meniscocapsular ligament are joined by the tendon's capsular

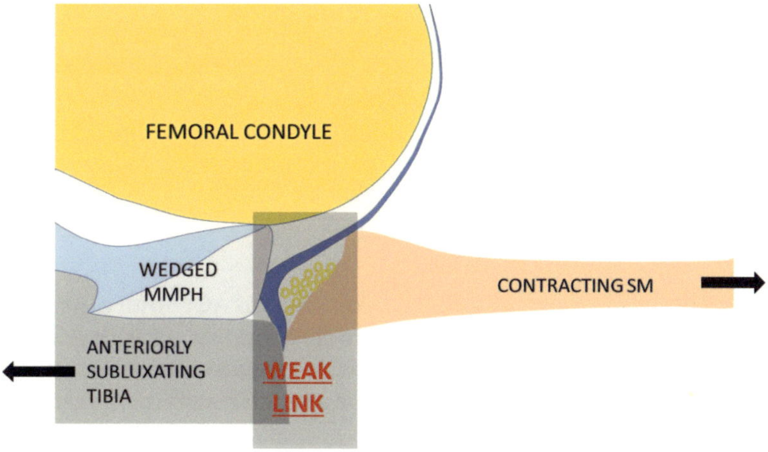

Figure 1.
Anatomy of the ramp.

limb, which connects to the medial meniscus's posterior horn. Ample adipose tissue with its own network of blood arteries was also found in this layer. This weak link is hypothesized to be the cause of ramp lesions. The well-vascularized nature might be implicated in the good healing potential of this region (**Figure 1**) [13].

3. Biomechanics

In addition to increasing anterior stability, the ramp area of the knee seems to aid in the joint's rotational stability [14, 15]. Medial meniscus longitudinal peripheral tear was associated with greater tibial anterior translation in ACL-deficient knees, as reported by Ahn et al. [16]. This improved significantly after the repair of such tears. However, there was no significant change in rotatory stability. According to Peltier et al. [5], there were no discernible changes in anterior translation between ACL-deficient knees, ACL-deficient knees with ramp lesions and ACL-deficient knees with a detached meniscotibial ligament. In ACL-deficient and ACL-deficient with detached meniscotibial ligament knees, internal and external rotation increased considerably under 5-Nm torque, respectively. After severing the meniscocapsular ligament, knees missing a posterior cruciate ligament were more prone to anterior translation and external rotation [17]. One additional clinical study [6] found a stronger correlation between combined ACL and ramp lesions and a grade III pivot test than between grade III pivot tests and isolated ACL tears.

4. Epidemiology

Most often, ACL tears go in conjunction with ramp lesions. Ramp lesions co-occurring with ACL tears have a frequency of somewhere between 9% [18] and 42% [19]. The incidence increase when the delay of ACL reconstruction is more than 3 months [20]. Jiang et al. [21] described 20 cases of ramp lesions over 2-year period without complete ACL tears. They noted ACL longitudinal splits in all these cases. They proposed that these longitudinal splits would have resulted in minimal anterior instability leading to ramp lesions due to semimembranosus contraction. Due to their invisibility on MRI and during arthroscopy [22, 23], the real prevalence of ramp lesions is unknown. These lesions may occur on their own or in conjunction with ACL tears. Ramp lesions have a same prevalence in both adults and children. Meniscal tears are more prevalent in children and teenagers; therefore, this is in sharp contrast to the general population [24].

5. Pathophysiology

The tibia shifts abnormally toward the front after an ACL injury. As a consequence of this stimulation, the semimembranosus muscle contracts, resulting in elongation of the capsular arm, meniscocapsular ligament and meniscotibial ligament. If the medial meniscus becomes trapped between the articular surfaces, a tear can develop if the ramp area gives way [13, 25, 26].

There have also been identified other ramp lesion development mechanisms. The most basic is the stress an ACL tear [27] places on the posteromedial joint capsule, which results in a valgus injury with internal rotation and axial loading of the tibia. A contrecoup injury can develop from a ramp lesion when the knee recovers from pivoting due to a varus strain and internal rotation of the femur on the tibia [28]. This technique results in a ramp rip in the medial meniscus by pressing it on the articular cartilages of the femur and tibia (**Figure 2**).

6. Clinical features

With these injuries, the anterior cruciate ligament (ACL) is frequently torn. Some of the clinical features that are indicative of the probable presence of ramp lesions include chronic ACL injuries of more than 3 months, a varus knee of more than 3 degrees [29], increased anterior tibial translation [18] and a grade III pivot test result [6]. A multivariate analysis of 769 ramp repairs found that ACL injury in the age group of fewer than 30 years had increased chances of developing ramp

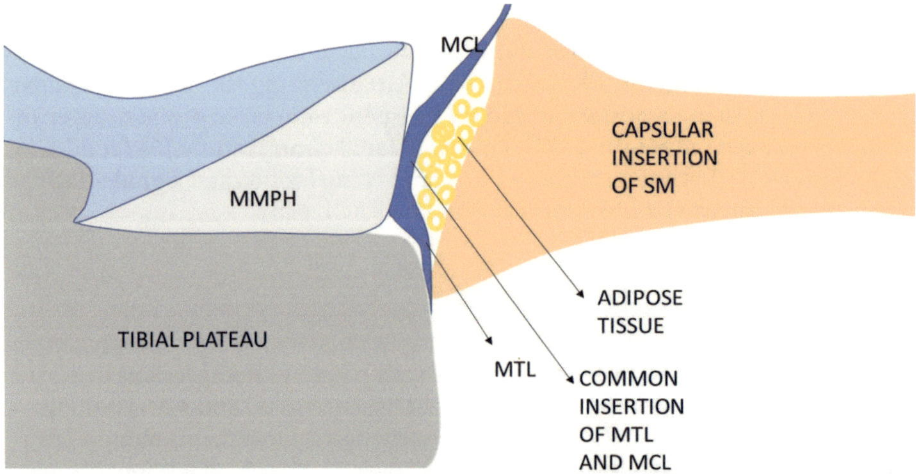

Figure 2.
Pathomechanics of RAMP lesion.

lesions. Males had 1.5 times increased risk of developing ramp lesions when compared to females. There is a strong correlation between the existence of a ramp lesion and a laxity difference of more than 6 mm from side to side [30]. A concomitant anterolateral ligament injury also increases the chances of ramp lesion [31]. Isolated ramp lesions, which are rare, present with posteromedial knee pain and pain on deep flexion [21].

7. Imaging diagnosis

On the other side, ramp lesions may be detected using the more common MR imaging of the knee. Injuries to ligaments and soft tissues may be treated with success using certain flexed-knee and/or 3D sequences (**Figure 3**) [22, 32].

Studies show that meniscal ramp lesions may be found using magnetic resonance imaging (MRI), which is both extremely sensitive and specific. Specificity was found to be 92–98% by Arner et al. [33], whereas sensitivity ranged from 53 to 84%.This sensitivity was observed by DePhillipo et al. [34]: The sensitivity and specificity of the meta-analyses and systematic review conducted by Koo et al. [35] were 71 and 94, respectively.

Hatayama et al. and Yeo et al. discovered that 3.0-T MRI was more capable of detecting ramp lesions than 1.5-T MRI [36]. By detecting an abnormality at the posterior border and complete fluid filling, ramp lesions may be accurately identified on MRI. While successive sagittal images may be utilized to pinpoint the damaged areas

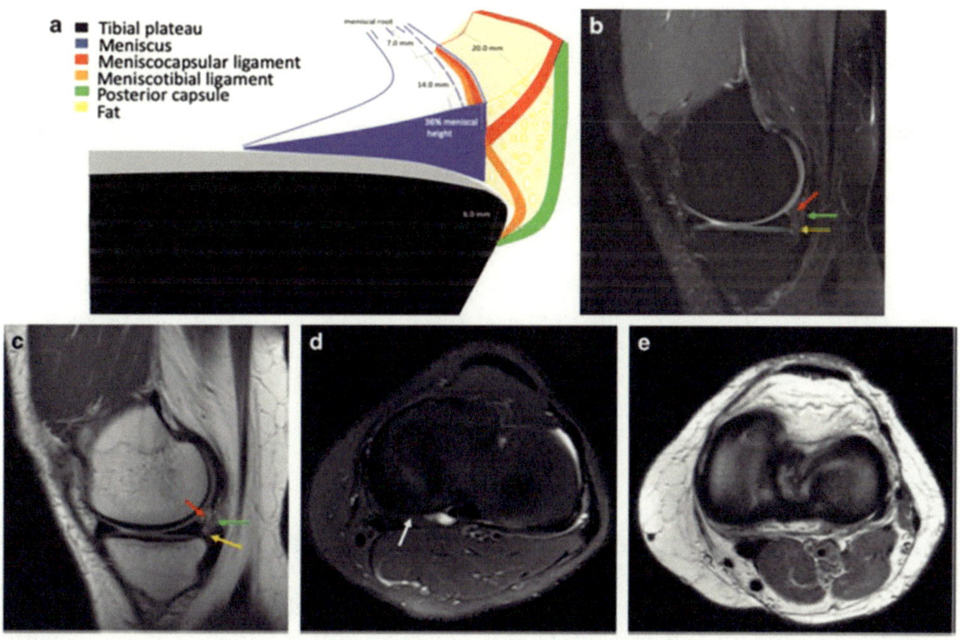

Figure 3.
a–e Normal composition. b. Any evidence of perimeniscal fluid separation was not seen during the sagittal proton density fat-suppression investigation. c. Fat signal intensity around the meniscocapsular junction is seen in a sagittal proton density image. Meniscotibial ligament, meniscocapsular ligament and posterior capsule (red arrow, green arrow) (orange arrow). d. Axial proton density fat saturation research found no evidence of perimeniscal fluid separation (white arrow). e. Proton density along the shaft.

	MRI findings pointing to the existence of a meniscal ramp lesion	**MRI results indicating an absence of a meniscal ramp lesion**
Primary findings	1. High T2 fluid signal intensity along the longitudinal, mediolateral, vertical and/or oblique axes, extending anteriorly, inferiorly or to both articular surfaces between the posterior horns of the medial meniscus and the posteromedial capsule. 2. Meniscocapsular attachment defects, which manifest as a localized discontinuity or a step-like contour distortion in the back of the knee, are caused by irregularities along the posterior margin of the medial meniscus. 3. Perimeniscal fluid's posteromedial corner of the knee's signal strength. 4. Soft tissue has grown between the medial meniscus and the medial collateral ligament.	1. Intact ACL. 2. When the red-red zone in the medial meniscus's posterior horn and the meniscotibial ligaments are present, the posteromedial meniscocapsular attachment is regarded as complete. 3. Medial and lateral meniscus linear T2 rips that do not impact the meniscotibial ligaments or attachments or extend past the red-red zone.
Secondary findings	1. Findings that indicate to simultaneous ACL damage: Tibial bone marrow edema with a posterior-medial distribution, consistent with a simultaneous contrecoup injury. • Transchondral fracture is found • The posterior cruciate ligament is harmed as a consequence of the lateral meniscus's back being exposed. • Utilizing a single coronal image to visualize the fibular collateral ligament • In relation to the lateral femoral condyle, the lateral tibial plateau grows forward.	1. No evidence of an associated ACL damage was found.

Table 1.
Summary of positive and negative findings for ramp lesions.

of the meniscocapsular junction and posterior horn, alternating sagittal and axial views can be used to assess the mediolateral and mediolateral dimensions of lesions [37, 38]. In **Table 1** we have compiled a summary of the MRI results, both favourable and negative.

8. Classifications

Meniscal ramp lesions have only been classified in the following few ways (**Table 2**).

- To evaluate whether a tear is adherent (self-heal) or dehiscent, adherent vs. dehiscent, and mediolateral vs. lateral, Seil et al. [39] analysed a set of cadaveric knees (repair).

- Instability, tear pattern, tear direction, tear thickness (partial vs. whole) and meniscocapsular disruption were all investigated by Thaunat et al. [40] in relation to meniscotibial ligament injuries.

DOI: http://dx.doi.org/10.5772/intechopen.112860

Thannaut et al.		Grief et al.	
Ramp lesions type	**Arthroscopic stability finding**	**Ramp lesions type**	**Arthroscopic stability finding**
Type 1: Meniscocapsular tear	Stable	Type 1: Meniscocapsular ligament tear	Stable
Type 2: Partial superior tear	Stable	Type 2: Partial superior peripheral meniscal horn tear	Stable
Type 3: Partial inferior tear	Unstable	Type 3A: Partial inferior peripheral posterior horn meniscal tear	Unstable
Type 4: Complete tear	Unstable	Type 3B: Meniscotibial ligament tear	Unstable
Type 5: Double tear	Unstable	Type 4A: Complete peripheral posterior horn meniscal tear	Unstable
		Type 4B: Complete meniscojunction tear	Unstable
		Type 5: Peripheral posterior horn meniscal double tear	Unstable

Table 2.
Classification systems in RAMP lesions.

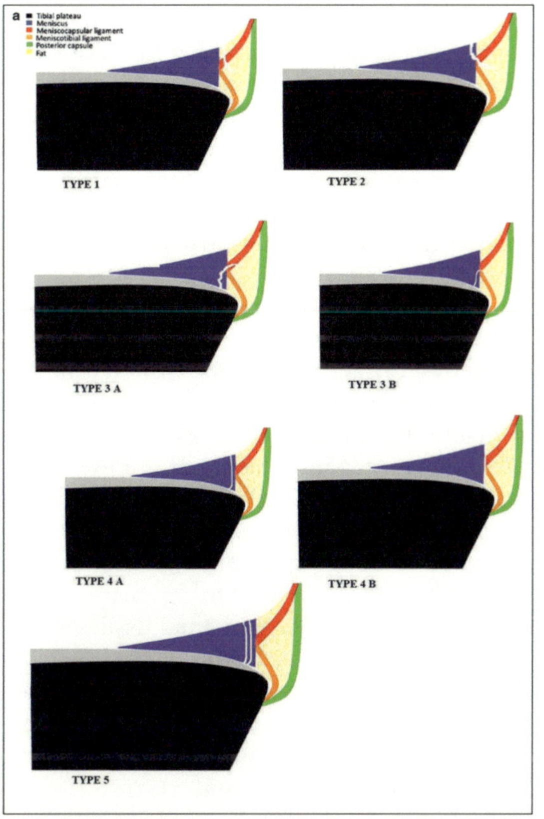

Figure 4.
Thaunat classification for ramp lesions.

- The Thaunat classification has been upgraded by Greif et al. [41] based on recent cadaveric investigations that support the union of the meniscocapsular and meniscotibial ligaments at the posterior horn meniscal connection (**Figure 4**).

9. Treatment

Meniscal ramp lesions have no consented treatment at the present time. Research has shown that ramp lesions in the context of acute ACLR may recover without surgical intervention if the surrounding biological conditions are appropriate. Some have suggested that ramp lesions should be surgically addressed rather than being let to heal on its own due to the hypermobility of the separated meniscocapsular component. There is data to suggest that individuals with similar longitudinal meniscal tear patterns who have ACLR without first having surgery may benefit from nonsurgical treatment. This is against the general view that ramp lesions should be addressed when there is chronic ACL insufficiency [16].

9.1 Repair procedure

For meniscal ramp lesions, when repair is the preferred therapy, the anatomic position of the lesion might provide a technical problem. The saphenous neurovascular bundle is at danger if a lesion in the posteromedial area of the knee is attempted to be treated. Repairing a ramp lesion requires careful attention to the saphenous nerve, therefore inside-out approaches should be utilized with caution and direct sight of the posterior capsule is preferred. Both inward-focused and outward-focused strategies have been effective in dealing with this issue. There is more room for movement when using sutures in an inside-out repair, which may lead to a more robust structure overall.

In the posteromedial technique for the inside-out repair, an incision is made vertically and obliquely from the adductor tubercle to the rear of the tibial plateau. The anatomical "triangle" formed by the medial gastrocnemius to the back, the inferior direct arm of the semimembranosus to the inferior and the anterior posteromedial joint capsule to the anterior may be seen after making a proximal incision in the soleus muscle fascia while keeping the pes anserine tendons *in situ*. The posterior neurovascular systems are shielded by a retractor while the wound is healing.

Using an arthroscopic self-delivery pistol with a cannula, double-loaded, non-absorbable sutures are placed into the meniscus in a mattress-like vertical pattern. The medial meniscal needle is placed into the upper or lower portion of the posterior horn of the medial meniscus with the knee flexed at an angle of 20 to 30 degrees. The meniscofemoral or meniscotibial capsule's opening is entered with the suture's second needle. Light pressure is used while clamping the suture ends. Another round of sutures, this time separated by 3–5 mm is used to complete the procedure. It is best to avoid putting too much weight on the posteromedial tissues while tying the meniscal sutures with the knee flexed at a 90-degree angle.

On the other hand, we may use methods that take place entirely inside the patient's body. While the advantages of these methods in terms of user friendliness and reduced neurovascular risks are undeniable, they are not without their share of drawbacks, including, but not limited to, discomfort from anchors, and meniscal body rips as a result of the larger holes formed by device insertion The stages of the repair procedure will be different depending on the tool.

However, there is currently no agreed-upon surgical rehabilitation programme for meniscal ramp injuries. Rehabilitation plans should start with broad concepts and be modified for each patient. In addition, when a meniscal ramp lesion and another knee injury occur simultaneously, the rehabilitation will be influenced in part by the simultaneous surgical operation.

10. Rehabilitation

Whether the meniscal ramp lesion treatment is an independent procedure or done at the same time as an ACL restoration affects the rehabilitation strategy. When an ACL reconstruction is done, the patient must undergo rehabilitation as outlined in the ACL rehabilitation protocol. On the first postoperative day, a patient who has undergone an isolated meniscal ramp repair should start performing exercises to reduce edema, improve knee range of motion, and develop the quadriceps. In the early postoperative phase, weightbearing and knee flexion are limited to minimise excessive stress on the repair. Maximum knee flexion activities (such as squatting and lifting) and pivotal and contact sports should be avoided for 4 to 6 months [42].

In average, patients who undergo repairs of tears to the outer two-thirds of the meniscus, such as ramp lesions, recover more quickly than those who have meniscal transplants or repairs of tears to the centre one-third of the meniscus. When a patient has a non-tender joint line, no pain or effusion, total muscle strength and full range of motion, particularly in full extension, they are prepared to resume sports or strenuous activities.

11. Conclusion

When it comes to ACL-deficient knees, ramp lesions are widespread yet sometimes ignored, especially in the acute situation. In ACL-deficient knees, these tears may induce substantial anterior tibial translation and external rotational instability, which can only be restored by performing a concurrent meniscal repair in addition to an ACL reconstruction. Ramp lesions are notoriously challenging to identify on MRI; hence, a thorough arthroscopic approach is often required for accurate diagnosis. Repairing ramp lesions is highly suggested if they are present to prevent negative biomechanical effects. Isolated ramp lesions should be treated with the same technique used for meniscal repair after rehabilitation as other knee injuries. However, if an ACL repair is done at the same time, recovery should adhere to the postoperative protocol for ACL reconstruction. Understanding about this injury type is essential, especially in the setting of an ACL tear, as ramp tears are more often than previously thought.

Author details

Iffath Misbah[1], Girinivasan Chellamuthu[2] and Munis Ashraf[3*]

1 Department of Radiodiagnosis, Saveetha Medical College Hospital, SIMATS University Thandalam, Chennai, India

2 Faculty of Research Karpagam Academy of Higher Education, Coimbatore, India

3 Department of Orthopedic Surgery, Saveetha Medical College Hospital, SIMATS University Thandalam, Chennai, India

*Address all correspondence to: munis6@gmail.com

References

[1] Hamberg P, Gillquist J, Lysholm J. Suture of new and old peripheral meniscus tears. JBJS. 1983;**65**(2):193

[2] Sonnery-Cottet B, Cruz RS, Vieira TD, Goes RA, Saithna A. Ramp lesions: An unrecognized posteromedial instability? Clinics in Sports Medicine. 2020;**39**(1):69-81

[3] Strobel M. Manual of Arthroscopic Surgery. New York: Springer; 1988

[4] Sonnery-Cottet B, Conteduca J, Thaunat M, Gunepin FX, Seil R. Hidden lesions of the posterior horn of the medial meniscus: A systematic arthroscopic exploration of the concealed portion of the knee. The American Journal of Sports Medicine. 2014;**42**(4):921-926

[5] Peltier A, Lording T, Maubisson L, Ballis R, Neyret P, Lustig S. The role of the meniscotibial ligament in posteromedial rotational knee stability. Knee Surgery, Sports Traumatology, Arthroscopy: Official Journal of the ESSKA. 2015;**23**(10):2967-2973

[6] Mouton C, Magosch A, Pape D, Hoffmann A, Nührenbörger C, Seil R. Ramp lesions of the medial meniscus are associated with a higher grade of dynamic rotatory laxity in ACL-injured patients in comparison to patients with an isolated injury. Knee Surgery, Sports Traumatology, Arthroscopy: Official Journal of the ESSKA. 2020;**28**(4):1023-1028

[7] Śmigielski R, Becker R, Zdanowicz U, Ciszek B. Medial meniscus anatomy-from basic science to treatment. Knee Surgery, Sports Traumatology, Arthroscopy: Official Journal of the ESSKA. 2015;**23**(1):8-14

[8] Taneja AK, Miranda FC, Rosemberg LA, Santos DCB. Meniscal ramp lesions: An illustrated review. Insights Into Imaging. 2021;**12**(1):134

[9] Yagishita K, Muneta T, Ogiuchi T, Sekiya I, Shinomiya K. Healing potential of meniscal tears without repair in knees with anterior cruciate ligament reconstruction. The American Journal of Sports Medicine. 2004;**32**(8):1953-1961

[10] Wymenga AB, Kats JJ, Kooloos J, Hillen B. Surgical anatomy of the medial collateral ligament and the posteromedial capsule of the knee. Knee Surgery, Sports Traumatology, Arthroscopy: Official Journal of the ESSKA. 2006;**14**(3):229-234

[11] DePhillipo NN, Moatshe G, Chahla J, Aman ZS, Storaci HW, Morris ER, et al. Quantitative and qualitative assessment of the posterior medial meniscus anatomy: Defining meniscal ramp lesions. The American Journal of Sports Medicine. 2019;**47**(2):372-378

[12] Benninger B, Delamarter T. Distal semimembranosus muscle-tendon-unit review: Morphology, accurate terminology, and clinical relevance. Folia Morphologica. 2013;**72**(1):1-9

[13] Cavaignac E, Sylvie R, Teulières M, Fernandez A, Frosch K-H, Gomez-Brouchet A, et al. What is the relationship between the distal semimembranosus tendon and the medial meniscus? A gross and microscopic analysis from the SANTI study group. The American Journal of Sports Medicine. 2021;**49**(2):459-466

[14] Papageorgiou CD, Gil JE, Kanamori A, Fenwick JA, Woo SL-Y, Fu FH. The biomechanical

interdependence between the anterior cruciate ligament replacement graft and the medial meniscus. The American Journal of Sports Medicine. 2001;**29**(2):226-231

[15] DePhillipo NN, Moatshe G, Brady A, Chahla J, Aman ZS, Dornan GJ, et al. Effect of Meniscocapsular and Meniscotibial lesions in ACL-deficient and ACL-reconstructed knees: A biomechanical study. The American Journal of Sports Medicine. 2018;**46**(10):2422-2431

[16] Ahn JH, Bae TS, Kang K-S, Kang SY, Lee SH. Longitudinal tear of the medial meniscus posterior horn in the anterior cruciate ligament–deficient knee significantly influences anterior stability. The American Journal of Sports Medicine. 2011;**39**(10):2187-2193

[17] Stephen JM, Halewood C, Kittl C, Bollen SR, Williams A, Amis AA. Posteromedial Meniscocapsular lesions increase Tibiofemoral joint laxity with anterior cruciate ligament deficiency, and their repair reduces laxity. The American Journal of Sports Medicine. 2016;**44**(2):400-408

[18] Tashiro Y, Mori T, Kawano T, Oniduka T, Arner JW, Fu FH, et al. Meniscal ramp lesions should be considered in anterior cruciate ligament-injured knees, especially with larger instability or longer delay before surgery. Knee Surgery, Sports Traumatology, Arthroscopy. 2020;**28**(11):3569-3575

[19] Balazs GC, Greditzer HG, Wang D, Marom N, Potter HG, Marx RG, et al. Ramp lesions of the medial meniscus in patients undergoing primary and revision ACL reconstruction: Prevalence and risk factors orthopaedic. Journal of Sports Medicine. 2019;7(5):2325967119843509

[20] Keyhani S, Esmailiejah AA, Mirhoseini MS, Hosseininejad S-M, Ghanbari N. The prevalence, zone, and type of the meniscus tear in patients with anterior cruciate ligament (ACL) injury; does delayed ACL reconstruction affects the meniscal injury? Archives of Bone and Joint Surgery. 2020;**8**(3):432-438

[21] Jiang J, Ni L, Chen J. Isolated meniscal ramp lesion without obvious anterior Cruicate ligament rupture. Orthopaedic Surgery. 2021;**13**(2):402-407

[22] Okazaki Y, Furumatsu T, Okamoto S, Hiranaka T, Kintaka K, Miyazawa S, et al. Diagnostic performance of open MRI in the flexed knee position for the detection of medial meniscus ramp lesions. Skeletal Radiology. 2020;**49**(11):1781-1788

[23] Peltier A, Lording TD, Lustig S, Servien E, Maubisson L, Neyret P. Posteromedial meniscal tears may Be missed during anterior cruciate ligament reconstruction. Arthroscopy: The Journal of Arthroscopic & Related Surgery. 2015;**31**(4):691-698

[24] Malatray M, Raux S, Peltier A, Pfirrmann C, Seil R, Chotel F. Ramp lesions in ACL deficient knees in children and adolescent population: A high prevalence confirmed in intercondylar and posteromedial exploration knee surgery. Sports Traumatology, Arthroscopy. 2018;**26**(4):1074-1079

[25] Qalib YO, Tang Y, Wang D, Xing B, Xu X, Lu H. Ramp lesion of the medial meniscus. EFORT Open Reviews. 2021;**6**(5):372-379

[26] Hughston JC. Knee Ligaments: Injury & Repair. 1993. pp. 300-315

[27] Young R, Devitt BM, Whitehead T. Meniscal ramp lesions: Diagnosis and treatment strategies. In: LaPrade RF, Arendt EA, Getgood A, Faucett SC,

editors. The Menisci: A Comprehensive Review of their Anatomy. Biomechanical Function and Surgical Treatment Berlin, Heidelberg: Springer; 2017. pp. 63-75

[28] Yoon KH, Yoo JH, Kim K-I. Bone contusion and associated meniscal and medial collateral ligament injury in patients with anterior cruciate ligament rupture. The Journal of Bone and Joint Surgery. 2011;**93**(16):1510

[29] Kim SH, Seo HJ, Seo DW, Kim K-I, Lee SH. Analysis of risk factors for ramp lesions associated with anterior cruciate ligament injury. The American Journal of Sports Medicine. 2020;**48**(7):1673-1681

[30] Sonnery-Cottet B, Praz C, Rosenstiel N, Blakeney WG, Ouanezar H, Kandhari V, et al. Epidemiological evaluation of meniscal ramp lesions in 3214 anterior cruciate ligament–injured knees from the SANTI study group database: A risk factor analysis and study of secondary meniscectomy rates following 769 ramp repairs. The American Journal of Sports Medicine. Nov 2018;**46**(13):3189-3197

[31] Ahn JH, Lee SK, Mun JW, Kim SW. Degree of anterolateral ligament injury impacts outcomes after double-bundle anterior cruciate ligament reconstruction. Arthroscopy: The Journal of Arthroscopic & Related Surgery. 2021;**37**(1):222-230

[32] Taneja AK, Miranda FC, Demange MK, et al. Evaluation of posterior cruciate ligament and intercondylar notch in subjects with anterior cruciate ligament tear: A comparative flexed-knee 3D magnetic resonance imaging study. Arthroscopy. 2018;**34**:557-565. DOI: 10.1016/j.arthro.2017.08.296

[33] Arner JW, Herbst E, Burnham JM, et al. MRI can accurately detect meniscal ramp lesions of the knee. Knee Surgery, Sports Traumatology, Arthroscopy. 2017;**25**:3955-3960. DOI: 10.1007/s00167-017-4523-9

[34] DePhillipo NN, Cinque ME, Chahla J, et al. Incidence and detection of meniscal ramp lesions on magnetic resonance imaging in patients with anterior cruciate ligament reconstruction. The American Journal of Sports Medicine. 2017;**45**:2233-2237. DOI: 10.1177/0363546517704426

[35] Koo B, Lee SH, Yun SJ, Song JG. Diagnostic performance of magnetic resonance imaging for detecting meniscal ramp lesions in patients with anterior cruciate ligament tears: A systematic review and metaanalysis. The American Journal of Sports Medicine. 2020;**48**:2051-2059. DOI: 10.1177/0363546519 880528

[36] Hatayama K, Terauchi M, Saito K, et al. Magnetic resonance imaging diagnosis of medial meniscal ramp lesions in patients with anterior cruciate ligament injuries. Arthroscopy: The Journal of Arthroscopic & Related Surgery. 2018;**34**:1631-1637. DOI: 10.1016/j.arthro.2017.12.022

[37] Yeo Y, Ahn JM, Kim H, et al. MR evaluation of the meniscal ramp lesion in patients with anterior cruciate ligament tear. Skeletal Radiology. 2018;**47**:1683-1689. DOI: 10.1007/s00256-018-3007-4

[38] Laurens M, Cavaignac E, Fayolle H, Sylvie R, Lapègue F, Sans N et al. The accuracy of MRI for the diagnosis of ramp lesions. Skeletal Radiology. Mar 2022;**51**(3):525-533

[39] Seil R, Hoffmann A, Scheffler S, et al. Ramp lesions: Tips and tricks in diagnostics and therapy. Orthopade.

2017;**46**:846-854. DOI: 10.1007/s00132-017-3461-z

[40] Thaunat M, Fayard JM, Guimaraes TM, et al. Classification and surgical repair of ramp lesions of the medial meniscus. Arthroscopy Techniques. 2016;**5**:e871-e875. DOI: 10.1016/j.eats.2016.04.009

[41] Greif DN, Baraga MG, Rizzo MG, et al. MRI appearance of the different meniscal ramp lesion types, with clinical and arthroscopic correlation. Skeletal Radiology. 2020;**49**:677-689. DOI: 10.1007/s00256-020-03381-4

[42] Chahla J, Dean CS, Moatshe G, Mitchell JJ, Cram TR, Yacuzzi C, et al. Meniscal ramp lesions: Anatomy, incidence, diagnosis, and treatment. Orthopaedic Journal of Sports Medicine. 2016;**4**(7):2325967116657815

Chapter 6

Anatomical Landmarks for Hamstring Tendon Harvesting in Anterior Cruciate Ligament Reconstruction

Radu Prejbeanu and Mihail-Lazar Mioc

Abstract

When performing an anterior cruciate ligament reconstruction (ACLR) with hamstrings autograft, one of the most delicate steps is graft harvesting. We will describe different anatomical landmarks that can be used in order to properly ensure that approach and tendon identification is facile. Knowing the anatomy of the 'pes anserinus' and different landmarks that can guide us towards harvesting is the goal of this chapter. Our descriptions will be based on existing literature and personal surgical experience. We shall also discuss different options described in the literature that have been used over the years. Knowing the correct anatomy as a surgeon helps improve our technique as such, we deal less local trauma and induce as little scar tissue as possible. Possible complications that can occur during the approach will be also discussed.

Keywords: hamstring tendons, pes anserinus, hamstring harvesting, ACL reconstruction, tendon insertions, tendon placement

1. Introduction

Tendon harvesting represents an important step during ACLR procedures. It is a step that, if performed properly can ensure a smooth surgical intervention. On the other hand, it is a step that can lead to different types of complications that can increase patient morbidity. Having good anatomy notions, helps us surgeons understand the functionality of the structures we see, and allows us to perform our interventions safely. Hamstring grafting especially, requires us to have good knowledge regarding the anatomy of the 'pes anserinus' and the muscles that are attached to it. We must also be aware of potential neurovascular structures that could be encountered during the graft harvesting procedure, in order to preserve them accordingly. The goal of this chapter is to ensure proper approach and tendon identification at the level of the 'pes anserinus' through the aid of anatomical landmarks. Intraoperative complications such as tendon slippage and neuro-vascular lesions may occur, and it is important to avoid them as possible or have functional solutions in case they appear.

2. 'Pes anserinus' anatomy

The 'pes anserinus' is a tendinous structure located on the antero-medial face of the proximal tibia. The tendons that make up the structures belong to 3 thigh muscles – the sartorius, the gracilis and the semitendinosus. These muscles act as knee flexors partial adductors and tibial rotators, counteracting the valgus stress of the knee. The sartorius originates on the anterior superior iliac spine and crosses over the anterior part of the thigh, whereas the other 2 muscles originate at the level of the ischial tuberosity (semitendinosus) and the pubic symphysis (gracilis). These 2 muscles, also known as hamstring muscles end in a very long, fusiform tendinous insertion, making them extremely good candidates for acting as donor sites for the ACL autograft.

2.1 Tendon insertions

The anatomy of the pes anserinus and its variations have been described by multiple authors [1–4]. Thus, it is important that we differentiate between the sartorius' tendon and the hamstring tendons (HT), as the first muscle has a thin and flat tendon, resembling a fascia layer, unsuitable for grafting [1]. The sartorius tendon (ST), gracilis tendon (GT) and semitendinosus tendon (STT) are united in a structure described as the *anserinus plate*. According to McMinn's illustrations, the ST is usually the most superficial structure and the GT and STT are usually situated deep and distally [5]. **Figure 1** depicts the pes tendons placement together with the local bony landmarks.

In a study published in 2019, Olewnik et al. described multiple anatomical variations regarding the structure of the pes anserinus tendons [6]. Regardless of the identified variation type, the ST is always proximal and superficial, and the HT are always deep and distal, as seen in the following schematic (**Figure 2**).

Even though roughly half (52.9%) of the analyzed knees presented with mono-tendinous insertions for each muscle, the authors also emphasize that the gracilis and the semitendinosus can often have accessory bands. Insertion variations such as short,

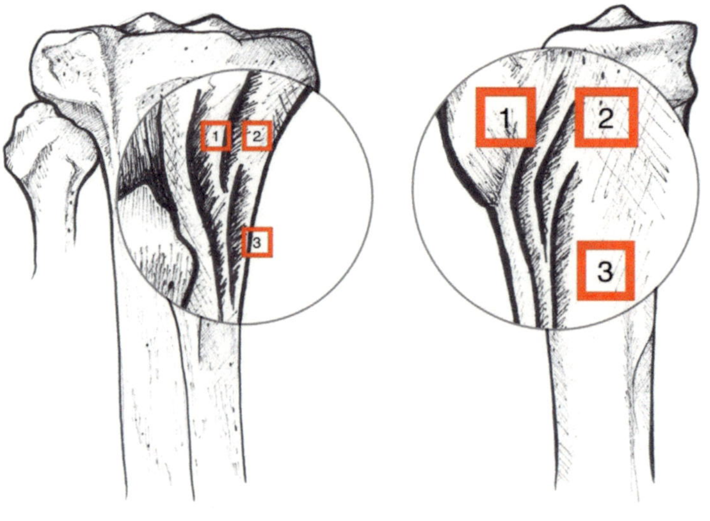

Figure 1.
Bony landmarks with ST (1) GT (2) and ST (3) insertions drawn out. Frontal view (left) and medial view (right).

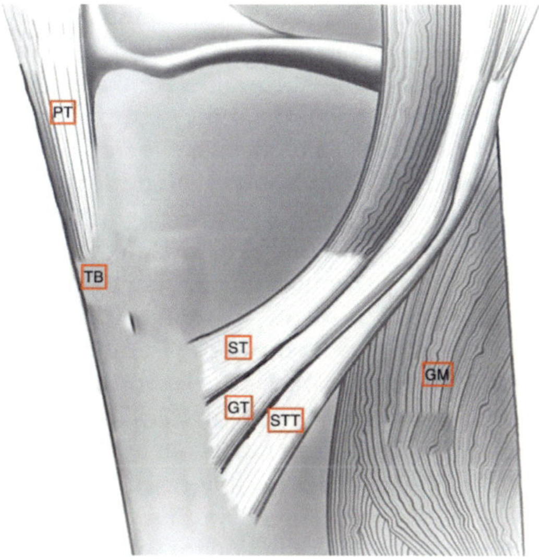

Figure 2.
Visual representation of the placement of tendon insertions on the pes anserinus (adapted from Olewnik et al.). (ST-sartorius tendon, GT-gracilis tendon, STT-semitendinosus tendon, PT-patellar tendon, TB-tibial tuberosity, GM-gastrocnemius muscle).

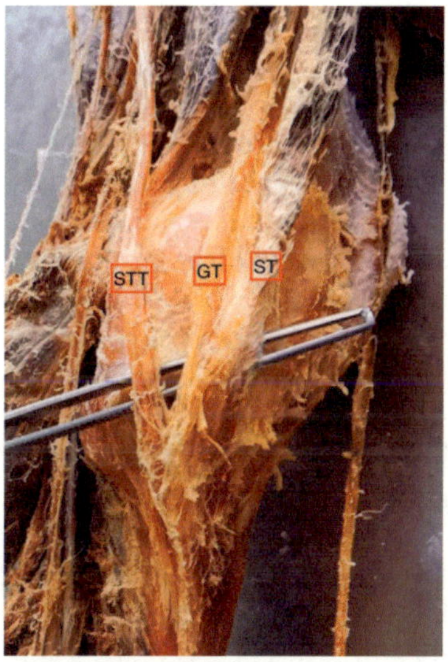

Figure 3.
Anatomical specimen depicting the 'pes anserinus. Poster-medial view of the knee. The surgical instrument is placed under the 3 tendons of the pes. From left to right we can observe the semitendinosus, gracilis and sartorius tendon.

band-shaped and fan-shaped can disorient the surgeon and lengthen the harvesting procedure [6].

2.2 Tendon placement

To further understand the local anatomy of the pes anserinus and the localization of the tendinous insertions, cadaveric studies [7] were carried out on fresh-frozen knees. The tendons are usually attached to the tibia on its antero-medial surface, through a conjoined structure that has an average width of 20 m. Warren and Marshall described two layers of the pes anserinus from superficial to deep in an older anatomical study. In the first layer we can find the sartorius tendon. It is superficial to the HT at its insertion and proximal part. Distally, we find it fused to the HT and as we continue into the deeper layer, we can observe that proximally and posteromedially they become distinct tendons. This specific point where the tendons become individualized is located on average 18 mm proximal to the conjoined insertion. Moving deeper, we can encounter the medial collateral ligament, that is situated in layer II [8]. This anatomical description helps us understand the local situation better and facilitates the isolation procedure of the two HT tendons.

Anatomical specimen dissections can clearly depict the placement of the tendon insertions on the pes anserinus as shown in **Figure 3**. The most anterior tendon is the sartorius, which quickly transforms into a muscle structure and is directed anteriorly over the thigh and laterally, representing the longest muscle in the human body. The other two deeper tendons belong to the gracilis and semitendinosus, they have a longer tendinous structure and are best suitable for ACL grafting. These two tendons are directed towards the medial and posteromedial aspect of the thigh.

3. External landmarks, incision and approach

Visual external landmarks play a big role in identifying the pes anserinus and aid in the initiation of the graft harvesting. Multiple studies suggest that the incision spot should be medial and slightly distal to the tibial tubercule. The usual technique describes the incision spot to be located medial from the tibial tubercule and 4–6 cm distal to the medial plateau (medial joint line). Lun et al. identify the starting point located 2 finger breadths below the medial tibial plateau, at the level of the tibial tubercule, extending distally [9]. This is often our preferred technique (**Figure 4**), as we take into consideration the medial tibial plateau, but we also place our incision taking into consideration the tibial tubercule solely. If measurements are done correctly, the position of the approach will coincide, regardless of the landmarks that were used.

The length and orientation of the skin incision do not matter too much as they play almost no role in influencing the identification of the tendon insertions. What it can influence though is the rate and severity of donor site morbidity and complications, that will be discussed later. Several authors describe different variants such as vertical and oblique incisions, ranging from 1.5 cm to 5.2 cm in length [10–17].

Performing the proper incision for HT harvesting may lower the risk of complications such as the iatrogenic saphenous nerve injury. This injury can cause symptoms such as hypoesthesia, anterior knee pain and reflex sympathetic dystrophy. The sartorial terminal branch and the infrapatellar branch are at risk when performing HT harvesting. The first could be damaged by the stripper, due to its proximity with the gracilis tendon, while the second may be damaged when performing vertical incisions in the approach of the pes anserinus. A systematic review performed in 2016 studied the complication rates of different types of incisions performed for HT harvesting [18]. It concluded that performing an oblique incision lowers the rate of saphenous nerve damage, when compared to either horizontal or vertical ones.

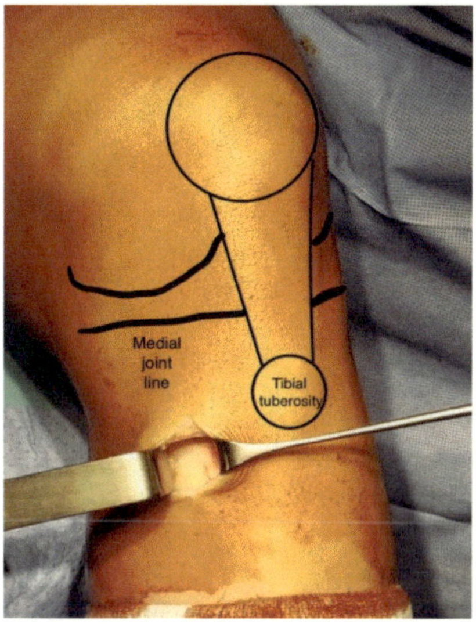

Figure 4.
Intraoperative photo of a left knee in a flexed position, depicting the approach we suggest for pes anserinus identification. Some key landmarks were drawn over.

4. Internal landmarks

As described previously, after the identification of the pes anserinus location, and performing the incision, we dissect the soft subcutaneous tissues to visualize the conjoined tendon of the pes anserinus. The current literature does not describe many subcutaneous landmarks that could help the surgeon.

There have been discussions regarding a vascular structure that can be encountered and could be used as an internal landmark. This vessel is a branch of the inferior medial geniculate artery (bIMGA) and is a part of the knee's superficial arterial grid. Some authors have depicted this vascular structure as a good indicator for pinpointing the insertion of the HT on cadaveric studies [9, 19, 20]. Babu et al. performed a prospective study on a lot of 100 patients, with a 98% rate of encountering the bIMGA during the approach. De Lima Lopes et al. performed ACL reconstructions on 30 patients and all of them presented a vascular ach at the level of the pes anserinus with "a greater or smaller diameter". Taking into consideration what these 2 manuscripts describe, allows us to believe that the bIMGA could serve as a proper landmark for the identification of HT insertion. The clinical relevance of it though, remains uncertain, as the amount of data is still small regarding this topic. There is also much to be discussed regarding anatomical variability and the ability of the surgeon to identify a small vascular structure through a small surgical approach. The reproducibility of the technique remains to be seen, as personal experience shows that there is a decently high variability, when it comes to encountering this vessel when performing the approach.

Proceeding through the skin and the subcutaneous tissue, we should be able to encounter the conjoined tendon of the sartorius, gracilis and semitendinosus. The two HTs are depicted in a surgical setting in **Figure 5**. Usually, the insertion of the gracilis muscle is proximal (superior) to the semitendinosus. Careful dissection of the conjoined insertion will lead to the identification of the two tendons which can then be separated, ligated and prepared for harvesting with either a closed or opened

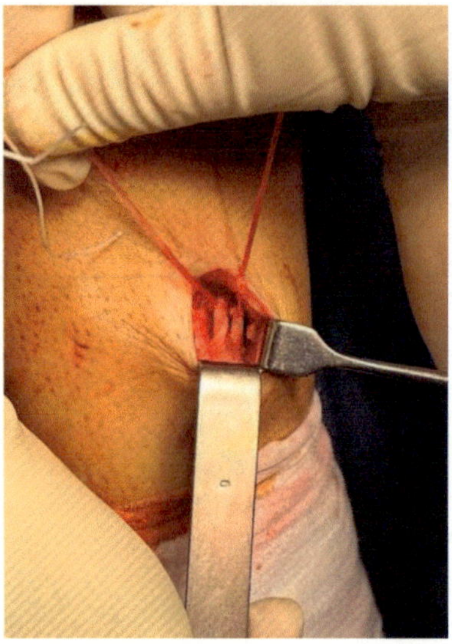

Figure 5.
Intraoperative photo of a dissected pes anserinus of the left knee. The two hamstring tendons can be observed – Gracilis tendon (left side) and hamstrings tendon (right side).

stripper. Special attention must be kept as to not mistake the sartorius insertion with the HT that usually lie distal and posterior.

5. Conclusions

Developing good knowledge regarding the anatomy of the pes anserinus helps the surgeon in the process of ACL graft harvesting. Young and unexperienced surgeons must take great caution in identifying the proper tendons and making sure that the harvesting process is done with as less trauma as possible. Even if complications may arise it is very important to identify them and address them properly.

Acknowledgements

Dr. Naomi Farcut – drawing Figure 1 pictures.
Dr. Lazarescu Adrian – providing Figure 3 from an anatomical specimen dissection.

Author details

Radu Prejbeanu and Mihail-Lazar Mioc*
"Victor Babes" University of Medicine and Pharmacy, Timisoara, Romania

*Address all correspondence to: mihail.mioc@umft.ro

References

[1] LaPrade RF, Engebretsen AH, Ly TV, Johansen S, Wentorf FA, Engebretsen L. The anatomy of the medial part of the knee. JBJS. 2007;**89**(9):2000-2010

[2] Ferrari JD, Ferrari DA. The semitendinosus: Anatomic considerations in tendon harvesting. Orthopaedic Review. 1991;**20**(12):1085-1088

[3] Lee JH, Kim KJ, Jeong YG, Lee NS, Han SY, Lee CG, et al. Pes anserinus and anserine bursa: Anatomical study. Anatomy & Cell Biology. 2014;**47**(2):127-131

[4] Candal-Couto JJ, Deehan DJ. The accessory bands of Gracilis and semitendinosus: An anatomical study. The Knee. 2003;**10**(4):325-328

[5] McMinn RM. Last's Anatomy-Regional and Applied. London: Churchill Livingstone; 1994

[6] Olewnik Ł, Gonera B, Podgórski M, Polguj M, Jezierski H, Topol M. A proposal for a new classification of pes anserinus morphology. Knee Surgery, Sports Traumatology, Arthroscopy. 2019;**27**(9):2984-2993. DOI: 10.1007/s00167-018-5318-3 Epub 2018 Dec 10

[7] Pagnani MJ, Warner JJ, O'Brien SJ, Warren RF. Anatomic considerations in harvesting the semitendinosus and gracilis tendons and a technique of harvest. The American Journal of Sports Medicine. 1993;**21**(4):565-571. DOI: 10.1177/036354659302100414

[8] Warren LF, Marshall JL. The supporting structures and layers on the medial side of the knee: An anatomical analysis. The Journal of Bone and Joint Surgery. American Volume. 1979;**61**(1):56-62

[9] Lun KK, Dan MJ, Broe D, Walsh WR. Inferior medial geniculate artery branch as an anatomical landmark for hamstring harvest during anterior cruciate ligament reconstruction. Arthroscopy Techniques. 2021;**10**(1):e177-e180. DOI: 10.1016/j.eats.2020.09.022

[10] Sanders B, Rolf R, McClelland W, Xerogeanes J. Prevalence of saphenous nerve injury after autogenous hamstring harvest: An anatomic and clinical study of sartorial branch injury. Arthroscopy. 2007;**23**(9):956-963. DOI: 10.1016/j.arthro.2007.03.099

[11] Luo H, Yu JK, Ao YF, Yu CL, Peng LB, Lin CY, et al. Relationship between different skin incisions and the injury of the infrapatellar branch of the saphenous nerve during anterior cruciate ligament reconstruction. Chinese Medical Journal. 2007;**120**(13):1127-1130

[12] Mahmood A, Nag H, Srivastava AK. Clinical and electrophysiological assessment of injury to infrapatellar branch(es) of saphenous nerve during anterior cruciate ligament reconstruction using oblique incision for hamstring graft harvest: A prospective study. The Knee. 2020;**27**(3):709-716. DOI: 10.1016/j.knee.2020.04.021 Epub 2020 May 11

[13] Joshi A, Kayasth N, Shrestha S, Kc BR. Infra patellar branch of saphenous nerve injury during hamstring graft harvest: Vertical versus oblique incisions. Journal of Nepal Health Research Council. 2016;**14**(34):180-185

[14] Keyhani S, Kazemi SM, Sajjadi MM, Elmi A. A comparison between oblique

and vertical incisions on the hamstring tendon harvesting in anterior cruciate ligament reconstruction and infrapatellar branch injury of the saphenous nerve. Revista Brasileira de Ortopedia (Sao Paulo). 2020;**55**(3):374-379. DOI: 10.1055/s-0039-1692695 Epub 2019 Aug 27

[15] Ochiai S, Hagino T, Senga S, Yamashita T, Oda K, Haro H. Injury to infrapatellar branch of saphenous nerve in anterior cruciate ligament reconstruction using vertical skin incision for hamstring harvesting: Risk factors and the influence of treatment outcome. Journal of Orthopaedic Surgery and Research. 2017;**12**(1):101. DOI: 10.1186/s13018-017-0596-x

[16] Mousavi H, Mohammadi M, Aghdam HA. Injury to the infrapatellar branch of the saphenous nerve during ACL reconstruction with hamstring tendon autograft: A comparison between oblique and vertical incisions. The Archives of Bone and Joint Surgery. 2018;**6**(1):52-56

[17] Sabat D, Kumar V. Nerve injury during hamstring graft harvest: A prospective comparative study of three different incisions. Knee Surgery, Sports Traumatology, Arthroscopy. 2013;**21**(9):2089-2095. DOI: 10.1007/s00167-012-2243-8 Epub 2012 Oct 17

[18] Ruffilli A, De Fine M, Traina F, Pilla F, Fenga D, Faldini C. Saphenous nerve injury during hamstring tendons harvest: Does the incision matter? A systematic review. Knee Surgery, Sports Traumatology, Arthroscopy. 2017;**25**(10):3140-3145. DOI: 10.1007/s00167-016-4217-8 Epub 2016 Jun 23

[19] Babu S, Gupte C, Gajjar S, Morris H. The 'sentinel' vessel: An anatomical landmark to identify the pes anserinus during hamstrings harvest for ACL reconstruction. European Journal of Orthopaedic Surgery and Traumatology. 2019;**29**(5):1115-1118. DOI: 10.1007/s00590-019-02408-4 Epub 2019 Mar 2

[20] de Lima LC, Arantes G, de Oliveira RV, Pinto DM, Gonçalves MC, Gonçalves RC. Anatomical reference point for harvesting a flexor graft during arthroscopic reconstruction of the anterior cruciate ligament. Revista Brasileira de Ortopedia. 2015;**50**(2):164-167. DOI: 10.1016/j.rboe.2015.02.010